Tone It Up

W9-BYM-853

Tone It Up

28 Days to FIT, FIERCE, and FABULOUS

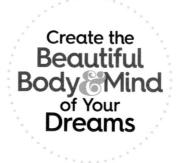

Create the
Beautiful
Body&**Mind**
of Your
Dreams

Katrina Scott & Karena Dawn
founders of Tone It Up®

RODALE

This book is intended as a reference volume only, not as a medical manual. The information given here is designed to help you make informed decisions about your health. It is not intended as a substitute for any treatment that may have been prescribed by your doctor. If you suspect that you have a medical problem, we urge you to seek competent medical help.

The information in this book is meant to supplement, not replace, proper exercise training. All forms of exercise pose some inherent risks. The editors and publisher advise readers to take full responsibility for their safety and know their limits. Before practicing the exercises in this book, be sure that your equipment is well-maintained, and do not take risks beyond your level of experience, aptitude, training, and fitness. The exercise and dietary programs in this book are not intended as a substitute for any exercise routine or dietary regimen that may have been prescribed by your doctor. As with all exercise and dietary programs, you should get your doctor's approval before beginning.

Mention of specific companies, organizations, or authorities in this book does not imply endorsement by the author or publisher, nor does mention of specific companies, organizations, or authorities imply that they endorse this book, its author, or the publisher.

Internet addresses and telephone numbers given in this book were accurate at the time it went to press.

To the Tone It Up community:
We are so grateful for all the love and support you provide for us
and for each other each day. You inspire us daily to keep living our dream
and continue to motivate others to live happy and fulfilling lives.

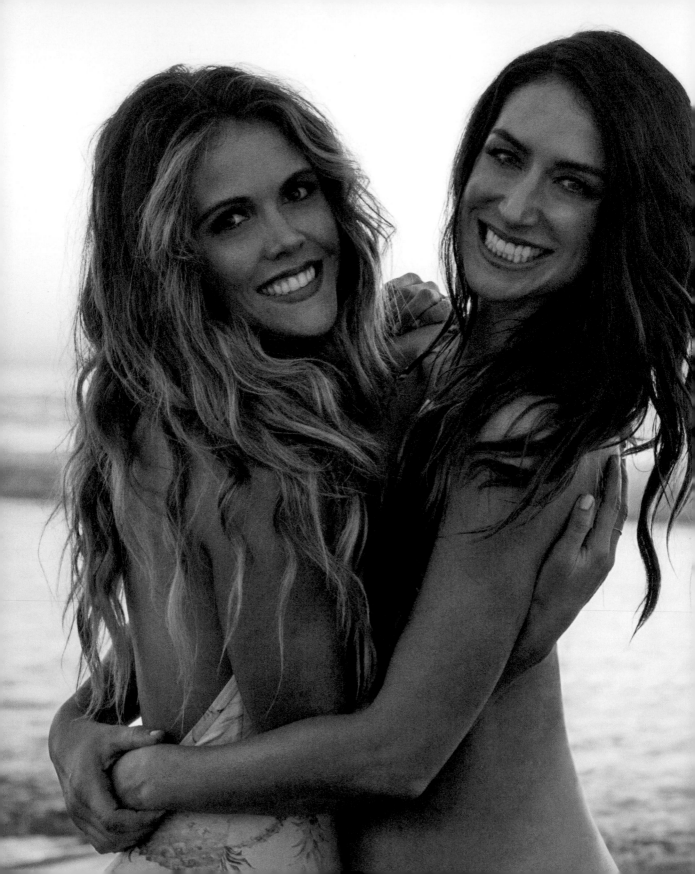

She's that girl you see with the UNMISTAKABLE something.

She's NEVER AFRAID to go after what she wants.

She TAKES CARE of herself, for herself.

She TONES her body, her mind, and her soul. Because she knows that if you're missing one, you don't really have the others.

She is BEAUTIFUL inside and out.

She works out because she LOVES HER BODY, not because she hates it.

She EATS HEALTHY FOOD. What she puts in her body is the fuel that powers her happy life.

She is the best girlfriend you could ask for: LOYAL, LOVING, up for anything.

She LAUGHS . . . A LOT . . . and never takes herself too seriously.

She doesn't dwell on the little things and knows how to LIVE in the moment.

She sets out to make a FANTASTIC life for herself every single day. She knows the secret to achieving happiness is to live it.

She stands tall with her shoulders back and heart open. She smiles. She is RADIANT because she knows how lucky she is to be strong and healthy and that she has the courage and tools to live her dreams.

She is FIT in body, FIERCE in mind, FABULOUS in life.

She is UNSTOPPABLE.

And in 28 days, she will be you.

Contents

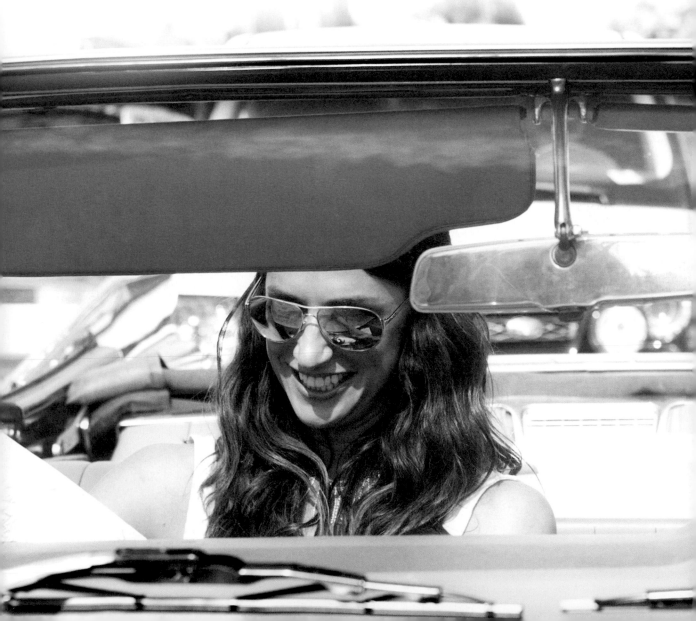

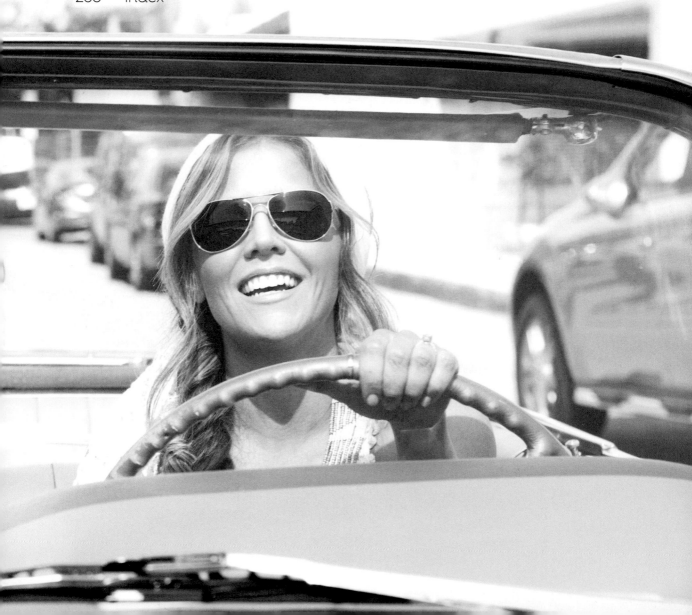

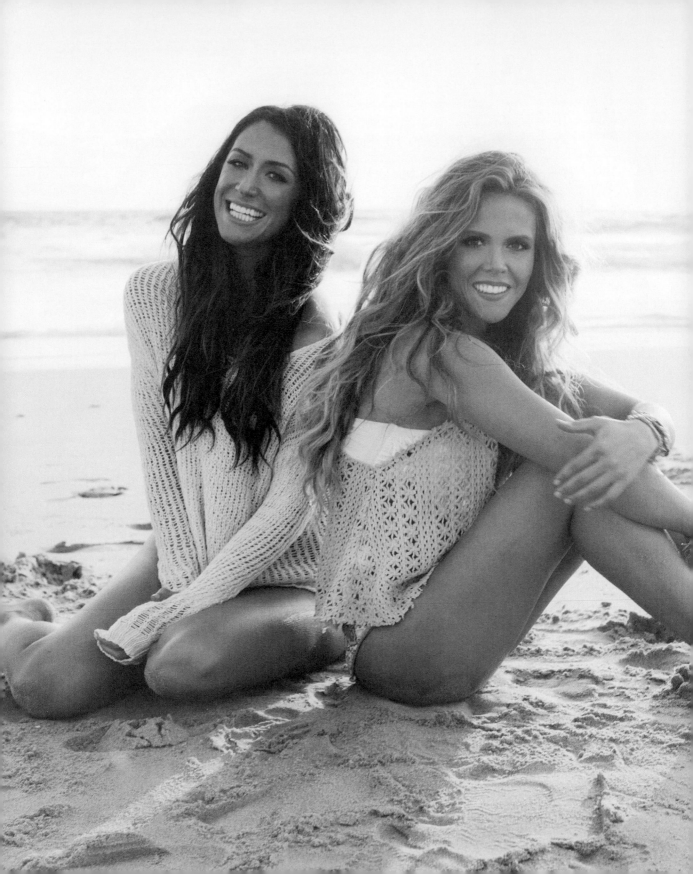

Introduction

Welcome, gorgeous gals, to our very first Tone It Up book. We're so thrilled you're here! Get ready, because the next 28 days are going to be a fantastic ride. You'll sweat, tone, nourish, empower, and laugh your way to your fittest, fiercest, most fabulous body and life!

Many of you already know us from our Tone It Up community. (Hi, TIU girls! How exciting is this?!) If you're new to our world, we're extra happy to have you, because you're about to discover some of the most inspiring friendships you can possibly imagine. Tone It Up is more than just a fitness brand; we're a worldwide community of strong, confident girlfriends who support each other in making our dreams happen and living exciting, happy, and healthy lives. But first let's back up a little so we can tell you how it all began . . .

In 2009 we were just two best friends with a vision. Both industry professionals—Katrina, a fitness instructor and

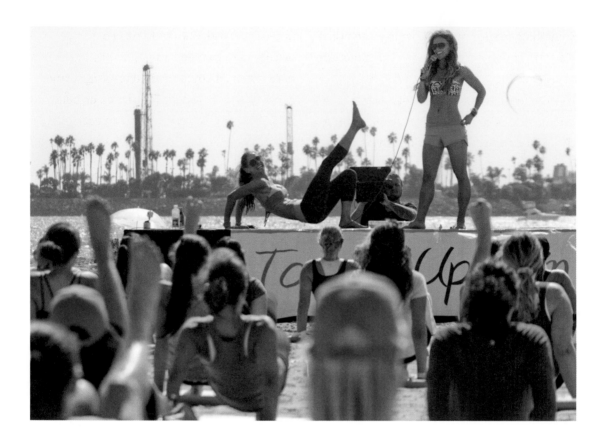

nutritionist, and Karena, a fitness model, triathlete, and spokesperson—we'd experienced firsthand the power of fitness to change our lives. We wanted to share that passion and create an active lifestyle brand that all women could relate to.

So with just a camera, two bikinis, and our determination in hand, we began filming homemade workout videos right on the beach near our Manhattan Beach home. (It was quite a process learning to work all the equipment. We'll admit it: More than once, we would film all day before realizing we forgot to turn on

the mics. Ouch!) When we put those first videos up on YouTube, we weren't sure if our audience was out there. But a few people tuned in . . . and then a few more . . . and a few more. It was happening!

Next we launched our "Tone It Up Meet-Ups," blasting out through social media a time and place where we were going to hold a free workout session, and women showed up—in droves! They would line up around the block with these beautiful smiles and infectious enthusiasm, and for 45 minutes we would sweat, stretch, lunge, and laugh together.

Something magical was happening. Each time was like a full-on fitness party with hundreds of like-minded girlfriends.

The most incredible part was how genuinely they were connecting with us and we were connecting with them. Every woman has a story when it comes to her body and self-care, and as we shared our personal struggles and experiences with them, they were opening up about everything from body image or food issues to difficult transitions they made and how fitness became their motivation (and outlet) for making real changes in their lives.

We felt honored to be trusted with so many of their inspiring stories. There was the mother and daughter team from New Jersey who each lost 70 pounds doing our workouts together; the circle of military wives in San Diego who banded together to tone up before their significant others came home from overseas (and to escape the loneliness that can be part of that life); the boyfriend of a Tone It Up girl who stood in line for 2 hours at one of our appearances just to thank us on behalf of his girlfriend and let us know how much the encouragement meant to her.

The sisterhood we'd lived in our own friendship was blossoming into a full-fledged community, with Tone It Up members connecting with one other—even without us. In cities around the country they would find each other through social media and meet up not just to work out but to hang out! It's usually hard to meet truly good girlfriends, but here it was all about women meeting women and creating real friendships based on building each other up rather than tearing each other down. We ourselves met through fitness, and by coming together to support one another, we were able to overcome personal obstacles and cheer each other on to follow our dreams. Just like us, these women felt that inspiring spirit of love and encouragement.

Given all this, we decided to take a leap. We quit our jobs and, living off our savings, set out to formally build our fitness company. We were so nervous! Could we really make a go of this? Would we succeed? Everyone thought we were nuts, but that didn't stop us. We went for broke—literally. What kept us motivated was having each other. Our deep friendship was cemented through all of the worry, late nights, long hours, challenges, and successes.

It was worth all the hard work. Today our videos have more than 35 million views. Hundreds of thousands of active Tone It Up members around the world are signed up for our newsletters, workout videos, and programs, and they link in with us through Facebook, Instagram, Twitter, and our online community (ToneItUp.com). We've had so much fun launching our Tone It Up health, beauty, and lifestyle gear, including our very own nutritional products company, Perfect Fit. But best of all, we wake up to thousands of women checking in with us about their workouts, posting recipes they love, and inspiring other Tone It Up members with their stories.

As you can see, it's been quite a ride! But the fun doesn't end there. We are writing this book to inspire millions more of you to become your most fit, fierce, and fabulous selves. We want to show you that you can create a toned body you feel confident in every single day; you can pursue your goals without fear or doubt; and you can live the sensational life you've always imagined. After all, if we did it, you can too!

Here's what you'll find in the pages to come . . .

In Part 1, "Becoming Fit, Fierce, and Fabulous," we'll share with you what it really means to be fit, to be fierce, and to be fabulous—Tone It Up–style! We take the meaning behind the words *fit*, *fierce*, and *fabulous* to heart and will challenge you to expand your view of each. We'll also share our own personal journeys to self-care and empowerment. It was a process of discovery and revelation for both of us, just like we're sure it will be for you.

In Part 2, "The When, What, and Hows of the Program," you'll find everything you need to know and do for the next 28 days. Throughout, we'll be right there next to you, every step of the way. We're your fitness BFFs, your guides on the path to phenomenal fierceness, and your fabulosity fairy godmothers, armed and ready with tons of motivational strategies, inspiration, body-changing moves, and beautifying tips for getting a gorgeous glow, inside and out. As a bonus, you'll also hear from some members of the Tone It Up community; we're all about sharing around here! And just to make sure you're set up for maximum success on the program, we'll also share our top five secrets for setting yourself up for the spectacular. Don't miss this important section!

Part 3 is our Knockout Nutrition Guide. We're here to help you build healthy habits for life, and that includes knowing how to make the best choices about how to fuel your body. In Part 3, we'll give

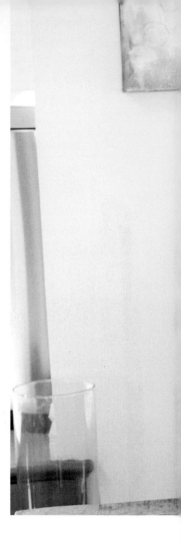

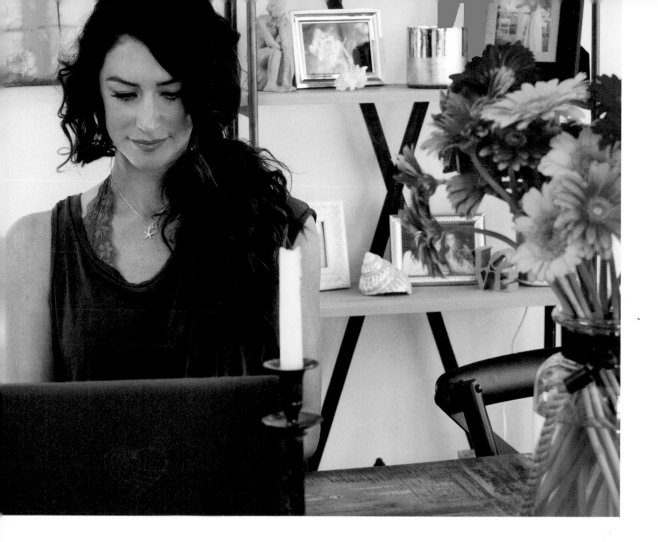

you our top 15 nutrition guidelines, the must-have essentials. Each day during the program, you'll also learn about a new superfood and recipe ideas to help you parlay these healthy eating habits into a permanent way of life. You can also find our official Tone It Up Nutrition Plan at ToneItUp.com. It's the perfect complement to this 28-day program!

Part 4, "Your 28-Day Fit, Fierce, and Fabulous Challenge," is the heart and soul of what you're here for: the program! You'll find your daily breakdown of what to do, divided into three sections: BE FIT, BE FIERCE, and BE FABULOUS. By the end of the very first day, you'll be well on your way to living and being all three!

Part 5, "The Workouts," is where you'll find the daily workouts and other exercises mentioned throughout the book. Each one is clearly explained with photos for easy reference.

Ready to get started? This is going to be a BLAST, beauties. Here we go!

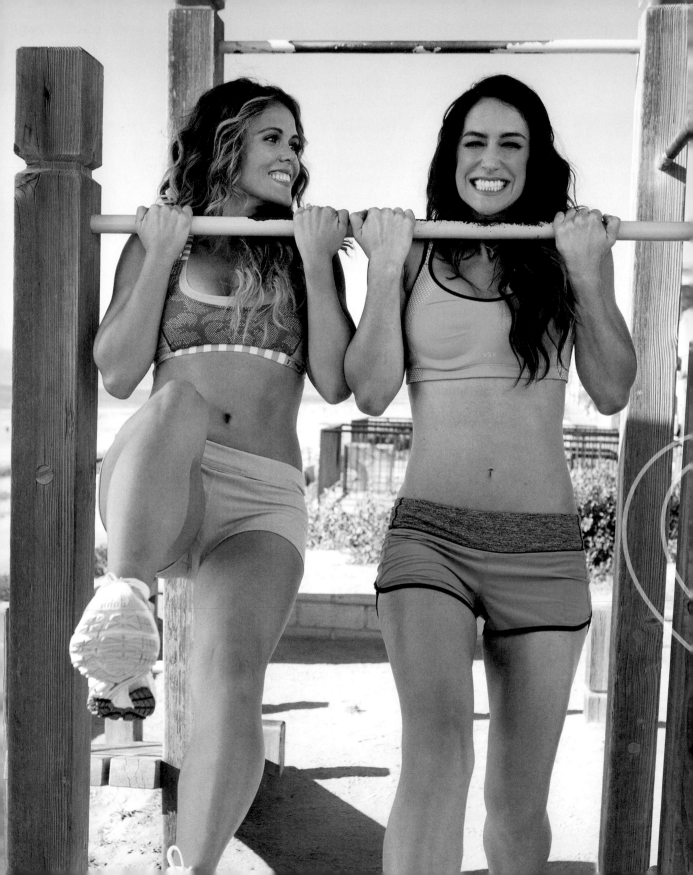

Part 1

Becoming Fit, Fierce, and Fabulous

Quick: What do you think of when we say the word *fit*? Having a toned booty? Killer abs, sleek arms, sexy legs? Absolutely, those are all part of what you get when you commit to being fit, and you'll achieve those (and more!) over the next 28 days.

But being fit goes way beyond looking smokin' hot in a bikini. Working out isn't just about vanity. It's about building confidence and how you take that into the rest of your life. True fitness is so much more than just the shape of your booty or the flatness of your abs, or even how fast you can run. It's a whole-body, whole-life way of being that comes from respecting your body and making the unshakable commitment to take care of your beautiful, amazing self, inside and out.

Being fit allows you to feel strong and sexy in your skin. When you're in shape and healthy, life is just so much sweeter, because you can be the spontaneous, always-ready-for-adventure babe that you are! You can do all the things you want to do in life, from dancing all night with your BFFs to trying a new exercise class you might never have dared to before. And let's not forget how much fun it is to be able to rock your favorite pair of jeans! When you're fit, you feel good expressing yourself in the clothes you wear, and as you know, that's a *big* deal for us as women.

In the days to come, through your BE FIT workouts and your new healthy eating plan, you're going to see some incredible changes in how you look. That's a promise! Your entire body will tighten and tone, and your skin will glow. But even more astonishing will be how you feel. You'll wake up with a clear mind and energy that's off the charts. You'll feel *fan-frickin'-tastic*, ready and raring to take on any challenge life throws your way!

The most amazing thing about fitness is how it transforms your mind-set. It ignites the fearlessness within you and empowers you to dream big and live boldly. You can flaunt, flirt, and freely express yourself. No more hiding, no more feeling self-conscious, no more hold-

ing back. Imagine the power in that! You may not know it yet, but you are a fierce lioness, filled with daring and confidence. All we need to do is awaken and unleash it! And that's exactly what you're going to do with the BE FIERCE Challenges in this program.

One last piece of the story is every bit as important as being fit in body and fierce in mind, and it is sparked by lighting up all the beauty that lives in your heart and soul. That's the essence of fabulous! Fun, friendship, laughter, creativity, generosity . . . these things give you that unmistakable glow. Being fabulous is all about taking good care of yourself and your inner universe so you can joyfully share your beautiful, loving, happy self with the world. With each BE FABULOUS Challenge you take on over the next 4 weeks, you'll become even more gorgeous and radiant.

Your whole life is about to change on every level. It starts with what you see in the mirror, then expands to how you feel and think about yourself, ultimately rippling out to how you light up from within and live your biggest, most fulfilling, most spectacular life. You're about to become a Fit, Fierce, and Fabulous goddess!

Our Stories

Neither of us just woke up one day and found ourselves living a Fit, Fierce, and Fabulous life. Just like you, this was something we had to make happen within and for ourselves! We've had our fair share of struggles with body image, confidence, and more, and we both discovered the power of fitness to transform our lives. We want to share our stories here with you, so you can see that when we say we get what it takes to make big changes from within, we REALLY get it!

Karena's Story

Fitness saved me. That's a bold statement, and it's really true. It showed me what I was capable of at a time in my life when I was convinced the answer was "nothing."

My teenage years were pretty rough. Life at home was complicated, and I kind of gave up on myself, on my career goals, and on the idea that I could ever accomplish anything. I found myself on an unhealthy path to self-destruction, eating crappy food and basically treating myself terribly. Seeking an escape from the anger and misery inside me, I turned to drugs. I'm far from proud to admit that I believed that magic mushrooms and ecstasy would deliver what their names implied. Of course they didn't, and I continued to search for the substance that would enable me to escape my reality, only to find myself digging a deeper hole. I may have appeared to be in good physical shape, but I certainly wasn't healthy on the inside, and my poor outlook and even poorer lifestyle choices showed in my dull skin and eyes that had lost their lus-

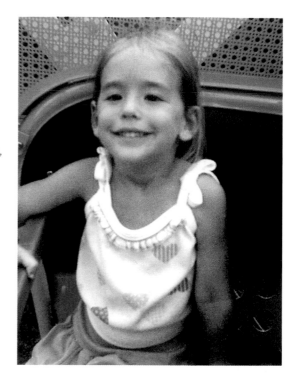

ter. The stress I was creating in my system eventually caused my body to break out in dry, flaky rashes all over. It was ugly and embarrassing, and I hid under layers so no one would see.

Eventually I found myself at a breaking point. After a doctor suggested I go to therapy and start doing yoga to relax, I got the message that I needed to make a change. I was unhappy and unhealthy, but I didn't *want* to be. I was tired of being depressed. I knew that I was facing one of only two choices: I could stay as I was and continue on this path to a life darkened by addiction and failure, or I could find the strength to overcome my past and break free of being a victim. Deep down, I knew I wasn't meant to give up on my life just yet. I finally got it that no one else had the power to make me happy or make me feel strong and confident; I needed to take control of my life and do it for myself. So I chose the harder route and began the work to free myself of the past and find the good life I was meant to live.

I thought back to the time in my life when I was happiest, as a kid, and what brought me joy. I'd always been interested in health and fitness, and I remembered running half-marathons with my dad and loving the feeling of freedom it gave me, so I decided to sign up for a triathlon. It was scary, for sure. I'd never pursued anything like that before with all my heart, because I'd always been sure I would fail, but I signed up anyway. It was make-or-break time, and I needed to prove something to myself.

It was intense and hard, and more than once I thought about backing out. Right up until the morning of the race, I was terrified. But I just kept telling myself, "You can do this. You're not a quitter anymore." No matter how much I didn't want to jump into the ice-cold ocean water, tie up my laces, or push through the last mile, I was determined. I knew that when I got through it, I would feel invincible. So I stuck to the promise I made myself and kept going—not without fear or doubt, but despite it. I overcame through the sheer act of doing.

I started crying when I crossed the finish line. In that moment, I knew I was beginning a whole new phase of my life. I finally believed I could *do* something. Scratch that: I finally believed I had the power to do *anything* I set my mind to!

After that, I started racing and competing in more triathlons. I got into personal training; began working as a sports and fitness model and an on-camera spokesperson for major

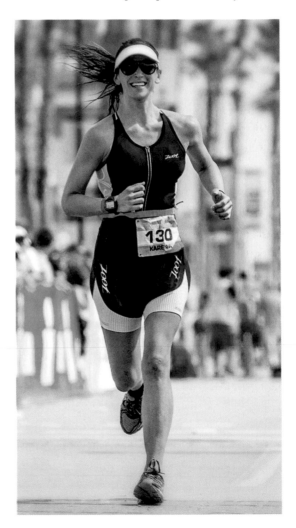

brands like Oakley, Adidas, and New Balance; and appeared in magazines like *Runner's World*, *Triathlete* (on the covers!), *Shape*, *Women's Health*, and *Self*. I found myself traveling the world, living this incredible life, doing what I loved. But I still knew there was more for me to accomplish. I wanted to use my life experiences to inspire other women to go after what they want and show them that—just like I learned—they're capable of anything and everything. I wasn't quite sure yet how I'd get there, but I knew that I would if I continued to believe in myself, do good work, and keep the vision of my dream alive.

In 2008 I moved to Manhattan Beach from nearby Marina del Rey after a tough decision to end a long-term love relationship. I was in a good place and excited about all the possibilities that might open up to me in this new phase of my life. That's exactly when Kat and I crossed paths. We discovered that we shared the same goals and dreams, and that first spark of "We can do something amazing together!" was lit. I'm going to let Kat tell you the rest of that story, so you can first hear everything from her end of what led her to that fateful, fantastic day when I met my beautiful, brilliant BFF and business partner!

Katrina's Story

Karena always says fitness saved her, and in a way I guess it saved me too—only under very different circumstances.

When I was 11 years old, I was about 20 pounds overweight. That was a pretty unhappy time in my life. I would hide on the sidelines at recess, watching everyone else having fun on the monkey bars and playing sports. If I tried to partake, they would literally laugh at me. No boys ever talked to me, and if they did, it was either to tease me about my weight or to ask me to deliver a note to my pretty and popular neighbor. I remember one girl telling me I wouldn't have any friends the next year in middle school because I was fat. I wasn't actually aware of the number on the scale back then. All I knew was that I couldn't wear the cute overalls that were in style at the time; the ones I'd bought hung in my closet, unworn. Let's just say they weren't that flattering on me, and deep down, I knew it. I didn't want to risk being laughed at any more than I already was.

I remember so clearly the day everything changed for me. I went shopping with my mom at 579, a clothing store specifically for juniors. As I was looking around, a saleswoman came over to us and said they didn't have anything there that would fit me. My mom was horrified. She'd always told me I was beautiful, and when the saleswoman implied that I was overweight, my mom looked at me with tears in her eyes, so worried that this woman had revealed something I didn't know. I knew my mom wanted to protect me, and it upset me to see her so sad about what had happened. But I'd known for a long time that I wasn't like everyone else. I went home that night and just cried and cried and cried. I was upset with myself and embarrassed that my mom had to witness what I went through every day with other kids at school.

But that fateful day was the turning point. I never, ever wanted to feel that way again, and I knew it was time to do something about it. The shame I felt that day turned out to be the motivation I needed to take control of my weight and health. Not for anyone else, but for my own confidence and happiness.

I started slowly, going for short runs in my neighborhood. Not long after, my dad asked if there was anything he could do to help me, and I had the answer ready: I wanted a treadmill and equipment to work out at home. My parents always supported me 100 percent in whatever I did, so my dad transformed our basement into a home gym for me. I ran every day and did exercise moves from fitness magazines. My grandma got me a nutrition book, and my mom let me start choosing the foods I ate. I lost about 15 pounds that summer, knowing that starting a new middle school that fall was my chance to start over. When I walked into the school that first day of seventh grade, kids from my old school barely recognized me. I went out of my way to talk to everyone and made lots of new friends. My newfound sense

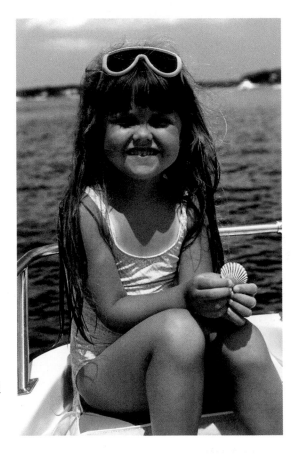

of confidence had profoundly changed me—and my life—for the better.

My interest in taking care of myself continued through high school, when I joined the tennis team, worked at a nutrition store where I learned all about vitamins and supplements, and started experimenting more with healthy cooking.

I knew I wanted to make fitness my life's work, so in college I studied health promotion and fitness, with a special focus on exercise physiology, sports nutrition, and training.

After graduating with my bachelor's degree in fitness plus every other certification I could scoop up in health and nutrition, I started working as a personal trainer in Boston. But it wasn't all smooth sailing from there. Sadly, my teachings and my habits weren't lining up, and I learned a hard lesson. I was so focused on my clients that I stopped focusing on myself, and in 1 year, I gained 26 pounds!

I started journaling to figure out what was going on. Journaling keeps us honest; it's easy to say "I'm healthy, I exercise," but when you write it down and see what you actually did and ate, things might look different than you'd imagined. I asked myself the same hard questions I'd ask my clients: "What is holding you back every morning from exercising, really and truly? Why did you make certain choices, like having an entire weekend of unhealthy eating? If you could do anything at all in the next 2 months, what would it be—and why aren't you living it now?"

That's when I saw I wasn't practicing what I was preaching. I would explain to my clients that if you eat junk food and skip workouts every weekend, you're making unhealthy decisions 12 days out of 30 each month; then I'd turn around and do that very thing to myself. I'd tell them to prioritize their morning exercise, then go ahead and book my schedule solid from 5 a.m. on, training clients and teaching classes so I had no time for my own workout. I was encouraging them to go after

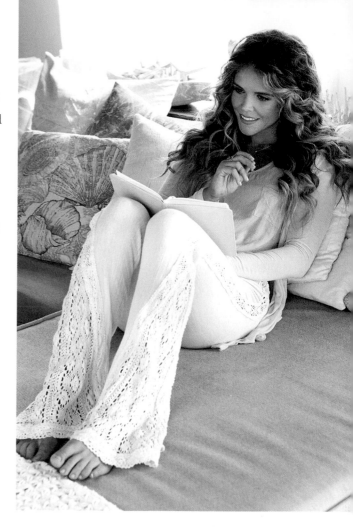

their dreams without fear, but I wasn't pursuing the big life that deep down I knew I wanted to create for myself. My vision was to make a living creating and posting fitness and cooking videos and inspire other women to take care of themselves and support one another. Seeing it all spelled out on paper was a big wake-up call, for sure.

After that, I recommitted to my health and well-being with all my heart and haven't looked back since. I moved with my then boyfriend (now hubby!) Brian out to California and started training clients and teaching classes in a much more sane, balanced way. I took the first steps to put my dream into action, posting some of my fitness videos on YouTube. I was cooking healthy food, exercising every day, and enjoying the beautiful, magical place I call home.

There was only one thing missing: Being new in town, I was a little short on girlfriends. After about the tenth time I asked Brian if my shoes went with my outfit or which necklace I should wear, he oh-so-patiently suggested I might want to find some other chicks to hang out with!

I'd see Karena come into the gym where I worked and always wondered what her story was. On some Friday nights she'd spend up to 2 hours working out or reading a book on the exercise bike. It was interesting to me that this beautiful girl was always by herself on weekend evenings, and I was curious if, like me, she was new in town and didn't know many people. I know it sounds kinda funny, but I just knew I wanted to be her friend.

One day at the gym, I finally went up to her while she was stretching and asked, "Do you do yoga?" Yup, that was my big pickup line! It felt a little awkward at first, but we started talking, and the girlfriend chemistry was just so immediate.

After that, Karena and I started running into each other everywhere we went: running on the boardwalk, at Trader Joe's in the organic produce section, at the local healthy eateries. Like-minded people tend to find each other because they hang out in the same places, and that was definitely true for us. Our orbits continued to intersect, and eventually we made some plans to take a yoga class together (it was my first, but I didn't tell Karena that at the time!). That led to morning walks together by the beach. We'd walk and talk, and quickly discovered we had the same big dreams and ideas, along with great synergy. I'd seen Karena's promotional videos on her Web site, and she was so

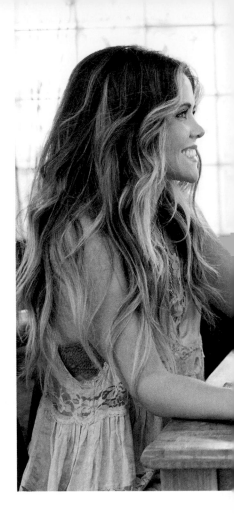

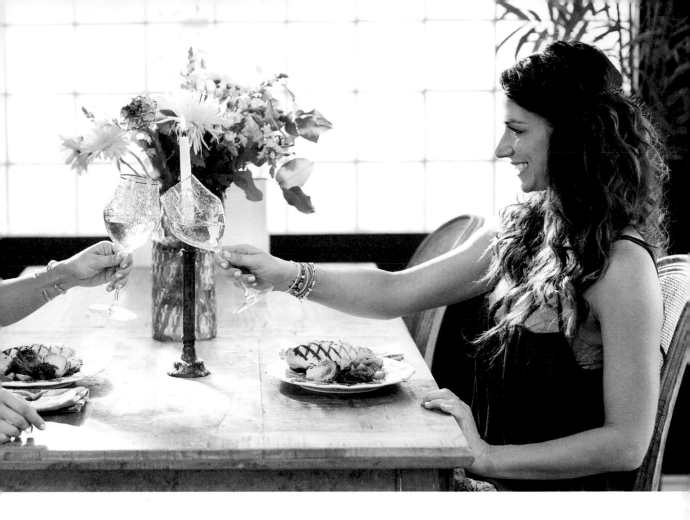

bubbly and warm on camera that I just knew that we could do something great together. So one day when I ran into her at Trader Joe's, I took a deep breath and just blurted out, "Let's film a cooking video together!" What was the worst thing that could happen? She'd say no.

Of course, by now you probably guessed that Karena said yes! Pretty soon we filmed our very first video in a friend's teeny-tiny kitchen and posted it. The viewers showed up, so we posted a few more. Then we did some

workout videos, and, well . . . you know the rest of the story.

Before Karena and I met, I had the fitness part down. She definitely had the fierceness. And when we met, that's when the fabulousness happened! We joined forces in friendship and partnership not just to inspire that in each other but in all of you. So now here we are, so excited to pass along all we've discovered so that you can become the Fit, Fierce, and Fabulous powerhouse we know you are!

Becoming Fit, Fierce, and Fabulous • **9**

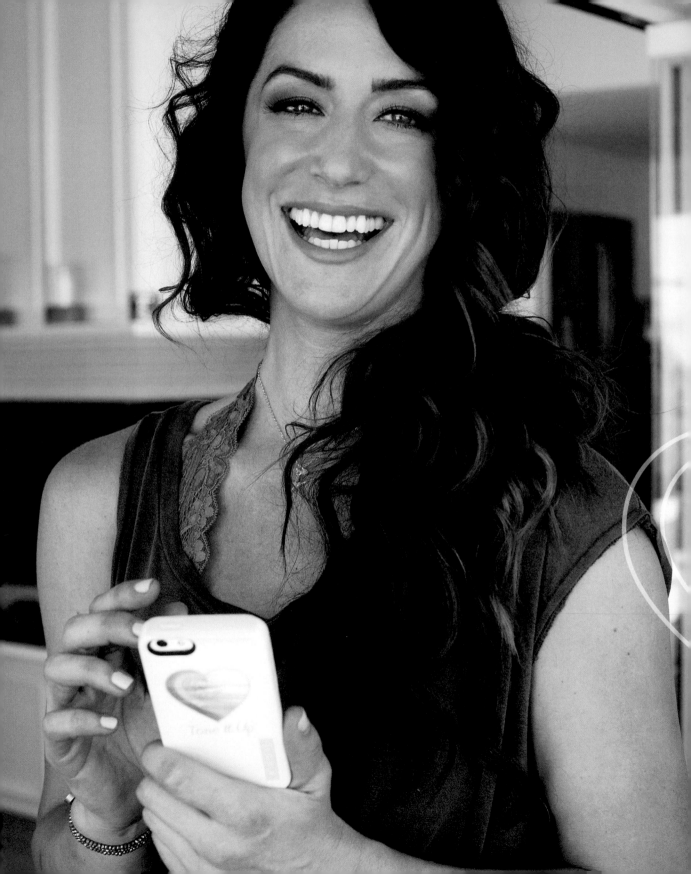

Part 2

The When, What, and Hows of the Program

Ready for the lowdown on the next 28 life-changing days? We want you to wake up on Day 1 ready and raring to go, fully armed with the info and inspiration you need to succeed big-time!

When?

Let's start with the obvious "when" question: "When should I start?" We arranged the daily program to begin on a Monday—the perfect morning for a fresh start of a new lifestyle! As you'll discover, the workouts and practices throughout each week are calibrated to the energetic pace of weekdays and more relaxed pace of weekends. So take out your calendar, mark the Monday you're going to begin, and be sure to read through all of Parts 2 and 3 between now and then to set yourself up for stellar success.

The second most important "when": "When can I expect to feel results?" The answer is right away, on Day 1. Yes, really! You'll be glowing with excitement generated by making yourself a priority, elated from the endorphins kicked up in your very first workout, and fueled with energy from the fresh nutrients you're loving your body with. Best of all, you'll feel empowered knowing you are well on your way to creating a whole new, healthy lifestyle for yourself. As the days zip by, you'll reveal sleek and sexy muscles, easily slip into your favorite jeans, and unleash your fierce fabulosity!

What?

As promised, we're here to guide you step-by-step through your daily routine. Here's every-

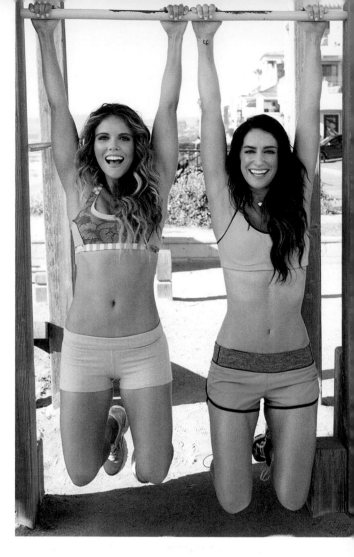

thing you'll be doing and discovering on each of the next 28 days:

Your Word for the Day

Motivated . . . gorgeous . . . joyful . . . strong . . . you are all of these things and more! Each day has a specific energy to it, captured by a single word. But these are far more than just simple words; each is your focus for that particular day, so take a pause sometime during your morning routine—even if just for a moment—to really take in its meaning. Each word will set the tone from the time you wake up until the time you go to sleep, to help you tap into all those fit, fierce, and fabulous qualities we know you want to magnify within yourself.

Your Daily Mantra

To keep the energy of the daily theme sparked throughout the day, we'll give you a mantra to say to yourself. We encourage you to write this mantra somewhere you can see it all day long, say on a sticky note on your bathroom mirror or in your phone as a reminder to ping you every hour on the hour. The power of suggestion on your subconscious mind is super strong, and we want to program that sexy brain of yours with all the positive stuff you're creating for and within yourself.

Your BE FIT Challenge

Let's face it: If you want to look and feel spectacular, you've got to get that beautiful body of yours moving and grooving and nourish it with the right stuff! BE FIT is the physical component of the program, and each day it includes:

- **Your Morning Booty Call.** Wake up, Sunshine—we're here to get you up and moving each day! Your Booty Call is the first of two workouts you'll do each day, but don't worry—it's meant to be short

and sweet, on average 15 to 30 minutes. It can be anything you like to do, as long as you're in motion: running, yoga, taking your pup for a long walk, even light stretching. Or choose one of the Fit, Fierce, and Fabulous Booty Call routines in Part 5. *Note:* If you prefer to do your longer Daily Fitness Challenge routine first thing in the morning, that's perfectly okay—just swap and do your shorter Booty Call later in the day or in the evening. The overall goal is just to make sure

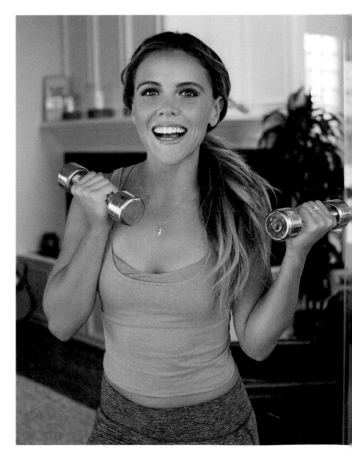

you're moving that gorgeous body of yours two separate times each day.

- **Daily Fitness Challenge.** This is your longer daily workout, which rotates daily. Each week you'll do two cardio routines, two power strength-training routines, and two high-intensity interval training (HIIT) routines, with one active rest day. As the weeks go by, the workouts get progressively more challenging, to keep your muscles guessing and your metabolism stoked. Throughout the program, in addition to your Daily Fitness Challenge, we'll sneak in lots of BE FIT bonus tips and tricks to sculpt your sexy, bombshell body.

- **Fab Food of the Day.** A superstar like you deserves super fuel, and we want to pack your diet with as many nutritional powerhouses as possible! To complement your Knockout Nutrition Tips, which you'll find in Part 3, each day we'll highlight one of our top 28 superfoods to get you lean, energized, and glowing.

- **Body-Loving Recipe of the Day.** We wouldn't leave you hanging without a fabulous way to put that day's superfood into use! From energizing smoothies to savory salads to decadent, healthy desserts, we'll arm you with tons of out-of-this-world delicious and easy recipes to try. We want you to have some fun with this; make trying new foods an adventure!

BOMBSHELL BONUS
Your Morning Motivation

We have good reason for getting you going bright and early each day. First and foremost: Consistency is key! If you make time for yourself first thing every morning, you're more likely to stick to your routine for the rest of the day. Plus, studies show that people who exercise first thing in the morning report better success burning off stubborn fat and losing inches. So set your alarm 30 minutes earlier every morning and commit to rocking this for the next 28 days!

Your BE FIERCE Challenge

You are a force to be reckoned with! Nothing is going to stop you from creating the body and life of your dreams, and we're here to make sure you rock this program—and every single day of your life after that.

Your daily BE FIERCE Challenges focus on your mind-set, to help you become your most confident, empowered self. Each day we'll give you a practice to keep you motivated and help you stay fiercely committed to your health and happiness. Some will ask you to step outside your comfort zone, but that's where the real change happens. We know you can do it!

Your BE FABULOUS Challenge

Ahh . . . time for some fun! Each day we'll give you a fabulosity-filled challenge to add some shine and sizzle to your life, ranging from a beauty indulgence to a fashion reboot to a frisky escapade with your girlfriends. *Please* don't overlook this essential part of the program; the joy and sparkle are every bit as important for your long-term glow as your daily sweat sessions!

How?

There's only one "how" that you need to know, and that's how you're going to make the magic happen!

We know it can sometimes feel overwhelming to get started. But that's why you have us! We're not just your trainers; we're your Fit, Fierce, and Fabulous guides, here to give you the tools you need to succeed and—even more importantly—a game plan to make sure you do.

We've had the privilege of training thousands of girls all over the world, and through our experiences and theirs, we've discovered the five secrets to setting yourself up for spectacular success. Follow these steps in preparation for your program and you can't miss.

Be Spectacular Secret #1: Get Organized

Like we said, on Day 1 we want you to wake up ready and raring to go—not frantically searching for your sneakers or scrambling to figure out what to make for lunch! Here's your checklist for getting organized:

- **Get your gear ready.** You'll need a high-quality pair of sneakers, a yoga mat or other form of exercise mat, a personal water bottle, and—if you don't have access to a gym—a set of free weights (we recommend one lighter set, from 5 to 8 pounds, and a heavier set, from 8 to 10 pounds). If you know you will want to do other activities for your cardio, get those ready to go as well (fill your bicycle

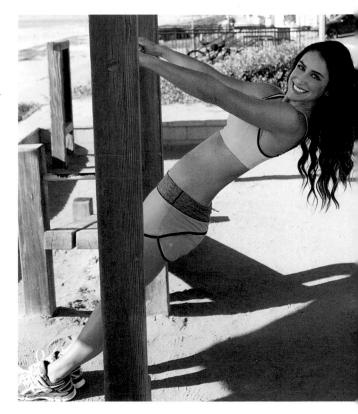

For a little extra motivation and inspiration, we created a Fit, Fierce, and Fabulous Tone It Up yoga mat and water bottle just for you! You can find it atToneItUp.com. xo K&K

tires with air, pull out your swim goggles, register for a 10-pack at your local spin studio, etc.).

- **Create a Fit, Fierce, and Fabulous Journal.** This can be a simple spiral notebook from the drugstore or a beautiful, bound journal with creamy pages or a Word doc on your computer. Personally, we like to use blank notebooks and decorate the cover with inspiring quotes and pictures, but it's up to you. You'll use this journal throughout the program for guided writing exercises, as well as to track your measurements each week (we'll guide you on when and how to do this).

- **Arrange your workout schedule.** At the beginning of each week on the program, map out your week's workouts in your Fit, Fierce, and Fabulous Journal. Don't just make a mental note of when you'll work out; actually schedule workouts in your planner or smartphone as commitments to yourself.

- **Plan your meals.** We're all for spontaneity, but not when it comes to meals! Plan out your menu for the following day the night before (especially breakfast). What will you have for meals? For snacks? Do you have all the ingredients you need? This is especially key for those of you who work in an office, because the lunchtime scramble or midday snack attack can blindside you if you aren't prepped ahead of time.

- **Read ahead.** This is important! Each day, make sure to read ahead to the following day's plan. You don't want to wake up in the morning and first read the Booty Call instructions then, because many days we suggest mental practices for you before you even step out of bed.

Be Spectacular Secret #2: Set Your Goals

What brought you here? Something motivated you to pick up this book and sign on for the next 28 days. What are you here to accomplish? Establishing concrete physical and emotional goals—and visualizing how you'll reach them (which you'll learn all about on Day 1)—is key to making your wishes into reality.

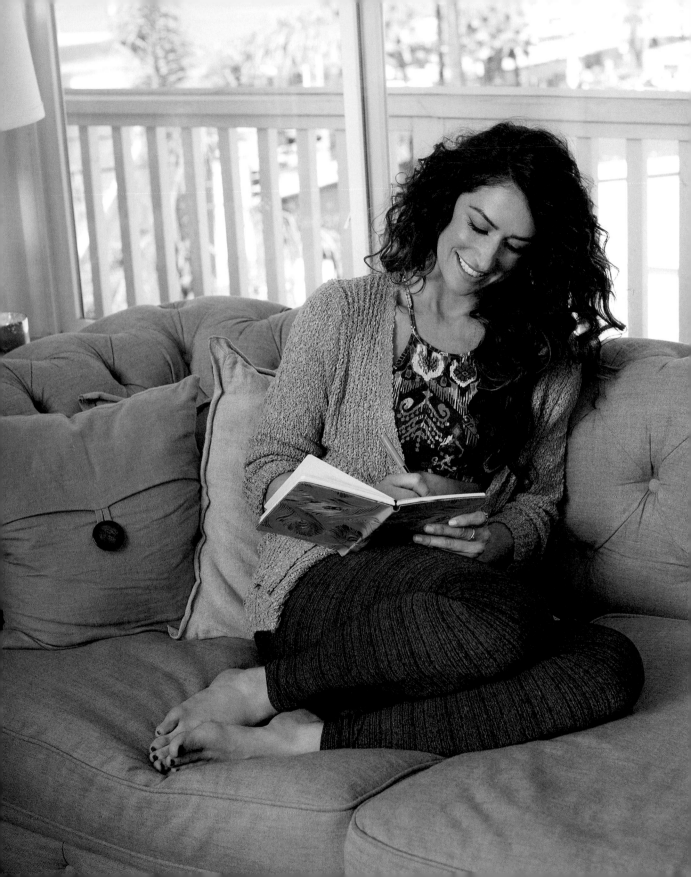

Here's your checklist for setting your Fit, Fierce, and Fabulous goals:

- **Write it to make it real.** In your new Fit, Fierce, and Fabulous Journal, write the answers to the following. Be sure to preface each with the words "I will" to get the manifesting muscles flexing and to write about what you *do* want (in the positive) rather than what you're trying to get rid of or get away from. We want those sparkling eyes of yours firmly fixed on where you're headed!

  My BE FIT Goals: Here are three specific things I want to achieve over the next 28 days in how my body looks and feels and how I care for my physical self (for instance, "I will feel stronger"; "I will rock short shorts"; "I will learn to prepare healthy meals for myself"): _____

  My BE FIERCE Goals: Here are three things I want to achieve over the next 28 days in what I believe about myself and what I can accomplish (for instance, "I will have the confidence to try new things"; "I will speak my mind"): _____

  My BE FABULOUS Goals: Here are three positive feelings and attributes I would like to manifest in myself over the next 28 days ("I will feel more joyful"; "I will have deeper connections with others"; "I will radiate!"): _____

- **Be honest with yourself.** Look over your list and do a gut check: Are all the achievements things you truly want, or do some just sound good? Sometimes we can be tempted to aim for what we think we should want, or for things that well-meaning others may want for us. But that doesn't mean they are particularly meaningful to *you!* Your goals should motivate and excite you and align with your innermost values. What does being your most fit mean to *you?* Your most fierce, your most fabulous? Dig deep: You and you alone know what you want to be, do, and have in life! Write down why each goal on your list is important to you and how you believe your life will be improved by reaching it. This will be a great reminder if you get off track.

Be Spectacular Secret #3: Track Your Measurements

Twenty-eight days from now, you're going to be toned, tightened, and TERRIFIC—and we want you to have the stats to prove it! As you're building and sculpting, you'll notice your waist getting smaller, your booty getting tighter and firmer, and your limbs becoming lean and sleek. We don't focus on weight; what matters more to us is what the measuring tape says and how your clothes are fitting. That's a much better gauge; you live in your clothes,

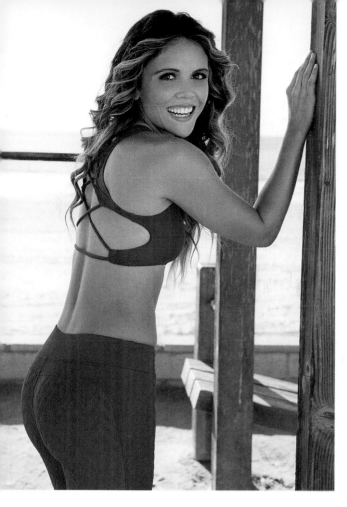

Hips/booty: Measure the circumference around the roundest part of your beautiful bum. (Damn, girl . . . that's a FINE booty you've got there!)

As you take and record these initial measurements, please: no judgments, no being mean to yourself, and definitely no feeling negative about what the numbers say. This is just data, and you're about to make some amazing changes! On the first day of each week, you'll retake these measurements (we'll remind you when) to witness yourself getting slimmer and tighter all over.

Be Spectacular Secret #4: Join the Tone It Up Community

If there is one core thing we're about, it's girlfriend power. We've not only seen the incredible results women get from having the support of other women (and encouraging them in return)—we've lived it ourselves. There are no girlfriends like the ones who share your passion for living healthy!

You already know we've got your back, but so do thousands of other Fit, Fierce, and Fabulous gals at ToneItUp.com. An entire community of ready-made girlfriends is out there waiting to support and cheer you on. The most unique thing about our community is there is zero negativity. It's all women supporting women, which is really refreshing. You'll find

not on the scale! Take the following measurements and record them in your Fit, Fierce, and Fabulous Journal:

- **Arms:** Measure the circumference of the place halfway between your shoulder and your elbow (where you see the sexy swoop of your triceps).

- **Waist:** Measure around your natural waistline, which is the smallest part, slightly above your belly button.

women talking positively about their bodies—and not being judged for it! They're proudly posting pics of their progress and getting applauded for it. If someone feels down about herself, the community lifts her back up. As you're becoming more fit, fierce, and fabulous, they will embrace all the positive changes you're making and encourage you to keep going.

But don't just take our word for it. Some Fit, Fierce, and Fabulous gals from the TIU community are here to tell you about their experience in their own words . . .

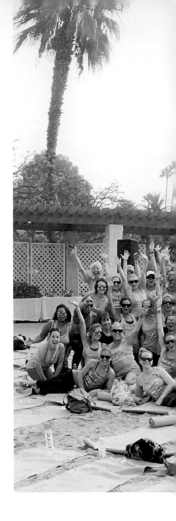

The women behind TIU inspire me daily. We all are battling something in our lives, and to see everyone strive for something greater is so inspiring.—**STEPHANIE F.**

Seeing all their check-ins from the girls in the TIU community motivates me to get my workouts done!—**KRYSTIE S.**

I am fortunate to have so many phone numbers of Tone It Up girls around the world that I can text or WhatsApp with at any time of the day and get a lovely response. Totally amazing. I LOVE that.—**PETRA S.**

In the last year and a half I have moved from Georgia to San Diego, to Houston, and now back to Northern California. Having the community every time I move has been life changing. I am beyond grateful for knowing that no matter where I go, I will always have amazing, inspiring women to meet up with!—**JULIA W.**

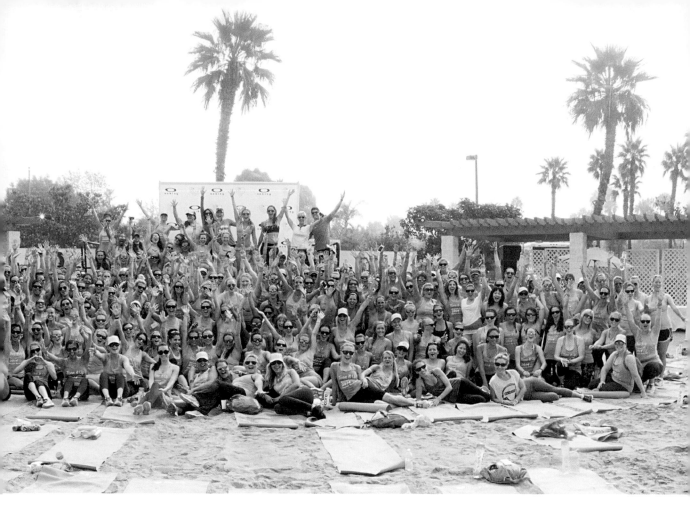

We are all so different from one another, but the common thread of Tone It Up creates an instant bond.—**JILLIAN M**.

I used to suffer from depression and feel very alone. I always struggled to lose weight, and nothing ever clicked. Meeting and talking to all the girls in the community really made me feel a part of something super special, and I no longer felt alone! There were thousands of girls just like me trying to accomplish the exact same goal . . . to be healthy! I found once I concentrated on being healthy instead of losing weight, that's when it really worked.—**JULIA M**.

The best part of being connected is that
I have thousands of girlfriends that understand
what I am going through. We are all on this
journey together.—**TIFFANY M.**

We're not just connected by wanting to look
good or run a 5-K—we share a love of life and fun
and spirit, and that's so special.—**KATY L.**

I have lifelong friends from all over the world
because of this TIU community. I am moving
from South Dakota to Arizona (1,600+ miles away),
and knowing there is a TIU group there makes
me feel relieved because I know I will make
friends right away!—**KARI B.**

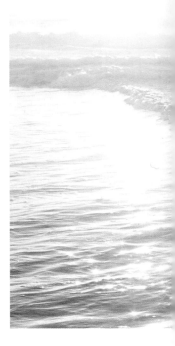

I initially started Tone It Up for the workouts and
recipes. I had no idea I would gain so much more.
I have literally made friends all over the
world. I have found and cultivated my passions for
working out, cooking, and treating my body like a
temple and I have also made the best of friends
along the way. The community is full of positive,
fun, uplifting, inspiring women. I am proud to call
these women my sisters.—**JENNY N.**

Pretty inspiring, isn't it?!

Besides the recipes, photos, and motivational stories you'll find
from hundreds of thousands of Tone It Up members, you'll find a special tab just for all of you on the Fit, Fierce, and Fabulous program.
You can also connect with others and share photos from your Fit,
Fierce, and Fabulous challenges by checking in on Instagram,

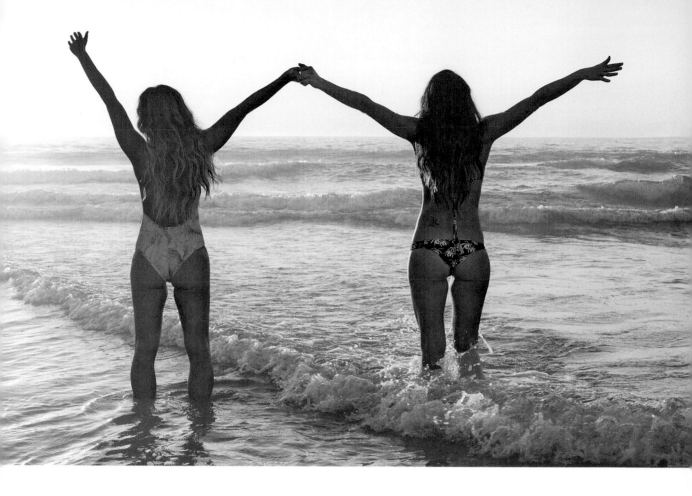

Twitter, Facebook, and in the Tone It Up community by using hashtag #FitFierceFab. You're not in this alone, sister—far from it! All you have to do is join the Tone It Up community to get tons of support, advice, and inspiration for your journey.

Be Spectacular Secret #5: Go for It!

You're ready. You're prepped. And in a very short time, you're about to put into action the plan that will enable you to create—once and for all—the body and life you've always dreamed about. So no holding back! Make a commitment to yourself, right here and now, that you're going to give this 100 percent. Everything you need to do is all laid out in these pages; that's our half of the bargain. All we ask is that you meet us halfway, with an open heart, shining eyes, and full willingness. Together, there's no stopping us!

Let's do it!

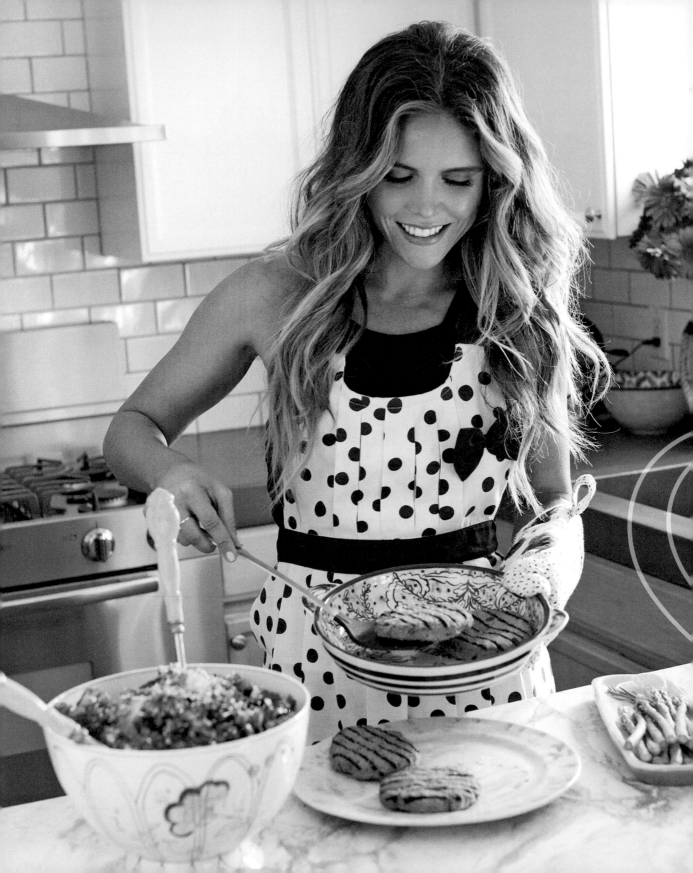

Part 3

Knockout Nutrition Guide

We're here to give you all the tools you need to become a bombshell babe, and that includes empowering you to make the best choices to nourish your beautiful body. This isn't about a 28-day quick fix. It's about adopting a whole new, lustrous lifestyle.

In the next few pages we'll reveal our proven tips for boosting metabolism and torching fat to reveal those sleek, sculpted muscles you're building. You'll learn how to make easy, healthy dishes, curb cravings, and keep your brilliant brain clear and sharp. Your energy will soar and your skin will glow! Incorporate these 15 Knockout Nutrition Tips into your daily

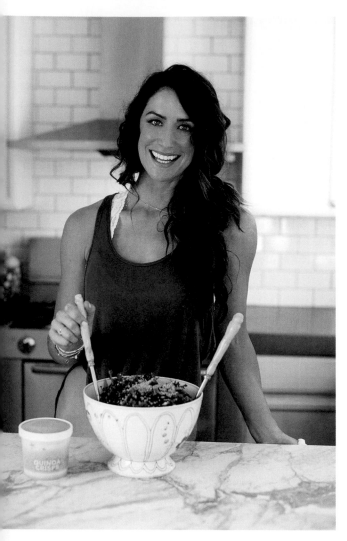

Knockout Nutrition Tip #1:

Get Fit with Fabulous Fiber

Fiber is a slim-down superhero, and we want you to include foods that are jam-packed with its potent powers at every single meal. Yes, you read that right: Every meal that you eat must include fiber! Why? Let us count the ways we love this fabulous phenomenon:

1. First and foremost: satisfaction, baby! Fiber is the ticket to feeling happy and full after eating a meal.

2. Fiber helps keep your blood sugar levels steady. Why should you care about blood sugar? Because that's what keeps us focused throughout the day, helps prevent cravings (bye-bye, uncontrollable grazing!), and enables our bodies to use the energy from our food efficiently.

3. Nearly all of the foods highest in fiber (think vitamin-rich veggies and fruits) pack a hidden bonus, which is clear, glowing skin. What you fill your body with on the inside shows up on the outside, and we want you to radiate!

4. Let's not overlook the health benefits! Fiber-filled foods keep your digestive tract in tip-top shape and lower your risk of heart disease, cancer, and other chronic diseases.

routine and you'll not only shed pounds—you'll gain confidence that is yours to keep forever, knowing you have the power to nourish your body to look and feel your best (and for an even more in-depth nutrition plan, you can also join our official Tone It Up program at ToneItUp.com).

Rock It Raw, Baby!

We love to snack on raw fruits and veggies; it's an easy way to get in vital nutrients and fiber, and it can make a huge difference in how you look and feel. Karena reaches for baby carrots for crunch and Kat loves sweet, fresh grapes. Unprocessed fruits and veggies in their most natural state are filled with enzymes that boost digestion and fight off disease, so we suggest reaching for whole, fresh, uncooked options whenever you can to ensure your body is power fueled, protected, and energized. Oh, and did we mention the raw-food gorgeous glow? It's real!

For fiber choices, think fruits, vegetables, legumes, and whole grains (for more on the best grains to choose, see Knockout Nutrition Tip #4). Fiber is naturally found in the cell walls of plants, so choosing more plant-based foods will automatically (and deliciously) increase your intake of fiber. Here's a list of our fiber faves:

Meet the Fiber Superstars

Artichokes (10 grams per medium artichoke, cooked)

Navy beans (9.5 grams per $\frac{1}{2}$ cup, cooked)

Edamame (8 grams per cup)

Lentils (8 grams per $\frac{1}{2}$ cup, cooked)

Raspberries (8 grams per cup)

Black beans (7.5 grams per $\frac{1}{2}$ cup, cooked)

Blackberries (7.5 grams per cup)

Canned pumpkin (7 grams per cup)

Chickpeas (6 grams per $\frac{1}{2}$ cup, cooked)

Chia seeds (5.5 grams per tablespoon)

Pears (5.5 grams per medium pear)

Broccoli (5 grams per cup, cooked)

Dried figs (5 grams per $\frac{1}{3}$ cup)

Sprouted grain bread (5 grams per slice)

Apple (4.5 grams per medium apple)

Avocado (4.5 grams per $\frac{1}{2}$ of an avocado)

Beets (4.5 grams per 2 beets)

Brussels sprouts (4 grams per cup, cooked)

Grapefruit (4 grams per grapefruit)

Oatmeal (4 grams per cup, cooked)

Almonds (3.5 grams per ounce)

Goji berries (3 grams per ounce)

Flaxseed (2 grams per tablespoon, ground)

Choose at least one of these fab-fiber foods to include in each meal every day, and we promise your waistline—and taste buds—will thank us!

Knockout Nutrition Tip #2:

Work with What Mother Nature Gave Ya!

In other words, just say no to fake foods. Besides interrupting your normal satiety signals (in other words, causing you to eat more), slowing your metabolism, making you feel sluggish, and dulling that radiant complexion of yours, the chemicals and additives in these foods cause you to hold on to stubborn fat cells that lead to hunger. We want you to say bye-bye to foods that are fried, processed, and full of chemicals, and in return you can say hello to killer abs, a healthy brain and joints, a lovely liver, spectacular skin, and a higher metabolism.

Chemicals in artificial sweeteners can also cause disease or unwanted side effects, so we're going to get rid of them for the next 28 days . . . at the very least! We know that once you experience how fantastic you feel without these in your system, you'll never go back. We understand if that sounds impossible right now to you; we ourselves used to be fake-sugar junkies. But those little devil packets can only hold you back from your goals— or worse. Take a look at Katrina's story on page 30 and you'll see what we mean.

Here are the foods we encourage you to steer clear of on your path to Fit, Fierce, and Fabulous:

- Any highly processed snack food (chips, store-bought cakes and cookies, etc.)
- Packaged "diet" foods (frozen dinners, fat-free cookies and candy, etc.)
- Anything that contains high fructose corn syrup. Read labels!
- Soda. Soda has absolutely no health benefits. In fact, it negatively impacts every organ it comes into contact with, from rotting your teeth to causing kidney problems. Diet soda is even worse, as it can mess with your metabolism. If the idea of giving up soda (diet or otherwise) sends you into a tizzy, fear not; just swap out the chemical stuff for the organic kind made with stevia. (Blue Sky is a favorite of ours.) We also like bubbly water flavored with natural lemon, lime, or berry.
- Artificial sweeteners such as Equal or Splenda and anything that contains them (like diet soda, sugar-free coffee creamers, and nonorganic fruit-laden yogurt). Stick to the real stuff. Stevia, coconut crystals, maple syrup, and honey are all Tone It Up approved! (For more on sweeteners and treats, see tip #13.)

You're probably now wondering, "Well, what *do* I eat?" We're so glad you asked. Mother Nature's pantry is where it's at! Eating nutrient-dense foods your body loves is essential for keeping your metabolism in

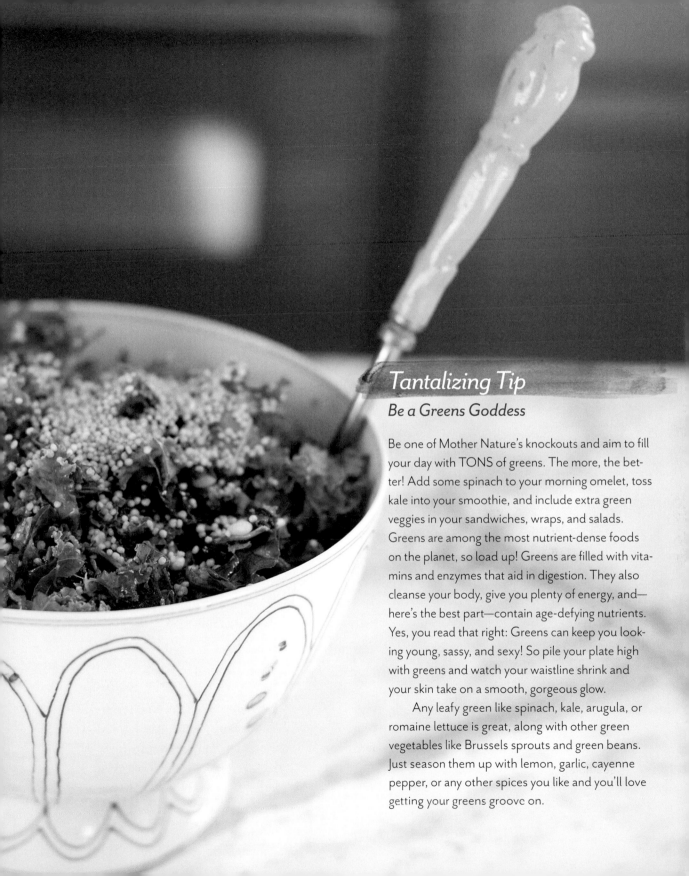

Tantalizing Tip

Be a Greens Goddess

Be one of Mother Nature's knockouts and aim to fill your day with TONS of greens. The more, the better! Add some spinach to your morning omelet, toss kale into your smoothie, and include extra green veggies in your sandwiches, wraps, and salads. Greens are among the most nutrient-dense foods on the planet, so load up! Greens are filled with vitamins and enzymes that aid in digestion. They also cleanse your body, give you plenty of energy, and—here's the best part—contain age-defying nutrients. Yes, you read that right: Greens can keep you looking young, sassy, and sexy! So pile your plate high with greens and watch your waistline shrink and your skin take on a smooth, gorgeous glow.

Any leafy green like spinach, kale, arugula, or romaine lettuce is great, along with other green vegetables like Brussels sprouts and green beans. Just season them up with lemon, garlic, cayenne pepper, or any other spices you like and you'll love getting your greens groove on.

Knockout Nutrition Bonus
A LITTLE LOVE FROM KATRINA

Here's Katrina's story about what inspired her to ditch the fake stuff—for good:

In my early twenties, I trained clients almost every hour of the day from 5 a.m. until 9 p.m. and taught a ton of classes and outdoor boot camps on top of that. As you already know from my story I shared earlier, even though I studied nutrition and knew how important it was to properly fuel my body, I was the last person I took care of. It was all about my clients for me.

In late 2007 I started having what my doctors referred to as mini seizures or blackouts. They were so scary. One time I was walking to dinner, and I fell to the ground and couldn't remember why I was there or where we were going. After a trip to the emergency room, I went for an MRI; I've never been so frightened. When they called to tell me they didn't find anything, I was relieved but also frustrated because the mini seizures continued.

That's when I started researching. Someone suggested I check my diet for aspartame and other fake foods loaded with chemicals. I thought to myself, "I'm healthy, I know what I'm doing, I don't need to change. Who are they to point to me as the problem?" But then I started writing down what I ate every day, and I saw that because of my go-go-go schedule, I was consuming all pre-prepared food and snacks. A typical day looked something like this:

5:45 a.m.: Iced coffee with sugar-free, fat-free creamer and a packet of Equal

7 a.m.: Protein shake with aspartame-sweetened protein. I didn't know it because it was at my gym café; but I investigated more, and sure enough, all the protein I was having had aspartame and count-less other chemicals I couldn't pronounce.

9 a.m.: Another coffee if I felt I needed it (okay, every day). More sugar-free creamer and an Equal.

11 a.m.: Grab a protein bar between clients. You bet it was sugar-free and loaded with chemicals.

1 p.m.: Lunch with coworkers. Salad with light dressing and a Diet Coke.

4 p.m.: Loved my light yogurt . . . loaded with aspartame, which of course I didn't know until I looked. I was just like the average consumer: too busy to check my labels!

6 p.m.: No time for dinner if I was still training! Another protein shake or bar from work.

9 p.m.: Home to another light yogurt if I wanted dessert.

In between all this, I had gum, flavored waters, and snacks that were supposedly "healthy." The common ingredient was aspartame. I cut out all aspartame and ate only whole, clean foods. Sure enough, I was cured!! I felt amazing . . . like I had overcome something that almost stopped me from living my life, training, teaching classes, or even feeling comfortable driving. Now I never touch anything with ingredients I can't pronounce. It scared me so much, I found the willpower to feed my body right, because I felt what it's like to start losing my health.

So you see, you can trust us when we say it's worth eating what Mother Nature made for you! She knows best.

high gear. Think lean proteins (like chicken, fish, quinoa, and tofu); fresh fruits and vegetables (especially greens; see page 29), nuts, beans, and legumes; whole grains; and natural forms of sugar like raw sugar, honey, and maple syrup. Bottom line: If it's found in nature, go for it. And as often as possible, choose organic sources of protein, fruit, veggies, and tofu.

For anything that comes in a bag, box, or other package, be sure to read the labels carefully; if you come across high fructose corn syrup; artificial sweeteners, colors, or flavors; or scary-sounding chemicals, run in the other direction as fast as those sexy stems will carry you. If you can't pronounce it, you probably shouldn't eat it. Unless it's quinoa. You should eat quinoa!

We want you to fuel your body with healthy calories and nutrients instead of chemicals. After all, if Mother Nature isn't the ultimate fit, fierce, and fabulous chick, we don't know who is!

Knockout Nutrition Tip #3:

Pack a Protein Punch

Protein balances your blood sugar levels to keep you satiated and wards off the insulin spikes that cause weight gain. Protein also keeps you lean, because it has a thermic effect on your body—or to put it another way, it

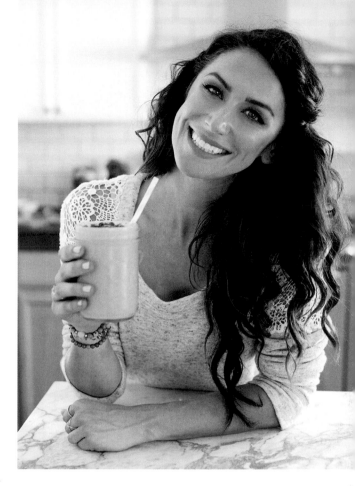

requires more energy to digest, so it helps your body burn calories.

Of course, we want you to pick the right proteins, and we're here to help you do just that. Here's your list of Fit, Fierce, and Fabulous–approved lean proteins. (Reminder: Opt for organic versions as often as possible.)

Chicken breast
Turkey breast
Grass-fed beef (limit this to once per week)
Fish
Scallops
Shrimp

Eggs (preferably egg whites; limit the yolks to one per day)

Greek yogurt

Almond, coconut, or soy milk (stick to no more than 1 cup per day, preferably in the morning, and make sure it's unsweetened)

Quinoa

Tofu (organic, non-GMO)

Tempeh

Legumes (beans, lentils, chickpeas, etc.)

Chia seeds

Hemp seeds

Spirulina

Perfect Fit protein powder

You want to include protein in as many of your meals and snacks as you can; four to five servings per day is ideal.

Knockout Nutrition Tip #4:

Choose Your Carbs Wisely

Carbohydrate has become a scary word in some circles, but not in Fit, Fierce, and Fabulousdom. We love carbs! They play a big role in keeping you lean and energized. Back in science class, you may have learned the phrase "Fat burns in a carbohydrate flame." Well, it's really true. Carbs are vital for burning fat. The trick is to choose the right kinds of carbs.

Just like you learned in Knockout Nutrition Tip #2, you want to avoid processed or packaged carbohydrates like crackers, chips, white breads, sugary cereal, white pasta, or candy. These will cause a sharp spike in blood sugar, which creates an energy burst–crash cycle that saps our energy and packs on the pounds. Additionally, these types of foods digest quickly, so they don't satisfy us for long. Instead of these processed carbs, experiment with nutrient-packed whole grains like whole oats, quinoa, amaranth, millet, brown rice, and barley. These are comforting, hearty, and filling and don't spike your insulin levels. And best of all, they give you the steady stream of fuel you need to power through your day—not to mention your workouts!

In the pages to come, you'll discover lots of tips and recipes for including these smart carbs in your daily nutrition plan.

Tantalizing Tip

Pick Protein for Postworkout Recovery

Whether it's cardio or toning, exercise breaks down your muscle fibers. To recover, you need protein, so make sure to refuel within 30 minutes of your workouts to replenish and get those sexy muscles of yours lean and sculpted.

Wonder Not

Remember that fluffy white bread from when you were a kid? Well, that spongy stuff is the exact opposite of fabulous. It's filled with chemicals and loaded with sugar, making you ravenous in the long run. Highly processed grains are stripped of their outer shell (the bran), which depletes the fiber that makes you feel full. Without the fiber, you're left with a substance that quickly turns to sugar in your body, leaving you hungry soon after you swallow that last bite. Choose whole grain breads instead (ideally from a bakery, rather than the packaged kind that tends to have lots of preservatives to keep it fresh on the supermarket shelves) to keep your blood sugar steady and your slender self satiated.

Knockout Nutrition Tip #5:

Go for the Good Fats

Like carbohydrates, good fats are nothing to fear. Fat gets a bad rap because . . . well, let's face it, it's called "fat." But *eating fat will not make you fat!* In fact, fats play a vital role in how we look, feel, and function. That is, if you eat the right fats. Those will keep your mind sharp (your brain needs essential fatty acids omega-3 and omega-6 to be in top form), your skin radiant, your mood elevated, your heart healthy, and your energy up. Good fats are also what make our food taste good and satisfy us, since they take longer to digest than carbs and protein and keep our appetite in check.

The types of fats we want you to incorporate into your diet are the polyunsaturated and monounsaturated kind. Choose from this list of our good-fat faves:

Extra-virgin coconut oil*

Avocado

Cold-water, fatty fish such as wild salmon, black cod, anchovies, and rainbow trout (and fish oil supplements)

Extra-virgin olive oil

Grape seed oil

Nuts and nut butters

Olives

Seeds

*While coconut oil is technically a saturated fat, its health benefits earn it a place on our good-fats list.

The fats we want you to avoid fall into two categories: saturated fats and trans fats. Saturated fats are mainly found in animal products like red meat and whole milk dairy products. That's why we encourage you to limit red meat consumption to once a week and ask you to stick to low-fat versions of yogurt. If you're a cheese lover (and really, who isn't?), it's perfectly okay to indulge now and then; just keep the portion size under control, as cheeses are high in saturated fat, calories, and sodium. The good news is that they do contain protein and calcium! Go for soft cheeses, which are generally lower in saturated fat. If you can, try to find a cheese that's made from fat-free milk.

Trans fats are nasty, evil stuff. There's a reason that California and New York City led the charge in banning the use of trans fats in restaurants and the FDA issued a warning against them! Trans fats are linked to heart disease, obesity, and depression. They are made with heated liquid vegetable oils and added to foods to keep them fresh longer (that explains the outrageously long shelf life of Twinkies!). Fast foods are usually loaded with trans fats, so steer clear of those. And read the labels on any packaged items you eat; if they contain the words *partially hydrogenated*, put them down and hightail it outta there. Those foods are ticking health bombs!

Knockout Nutrition Tip #6:
Be a Breakfast Believer

The big B is nonnegotiable, chiquitas! It's an essential part of your Fit, Fierce, and Fabulous lifestyle. Here's why:

A power boost in the morning starts your day off right. It kick-starts your metabolism and gives you a healthy burst of energy, which in turn makes you much more productive. It's a mental motivational boost, as it signals your brain and body that today is going to be a glowing, gorgeous day, fueled by healthy food and practices. Lastly, it sets you up to make good choices for the rest of the day. Skipping that morning meal ensures you'll be hungry later, which makes you more prone to cravings and un-fab food pitfalls.

Choose a protein-filled breakfast like one of these options:

Tantalizing Tip
Forgo Fake "Fat-Free" Foods

While we're on the topic of fats, if anything other than fresh food claims to be "fat-free," just know that is code for "crammed with chemicals." Those fake, fat-free sweets and snacks can never satisfy you the way real food can. Plus, they taste awful!

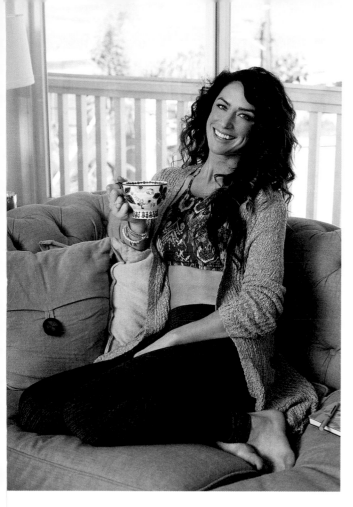

- Plain Greek yogurt (0%–1% fat) with fruit or low-sugar granola

- Egg white omelet with veggies (or make it into a whole wheat wrap)

- Oatmeal (whole, not instant) with fruit and ¼ cup almonds

- Our Perfect Fit Pancakes. Yes, you heard that right: pancakes! This is a Tone It Up Nutrition Plan favorite, and the recipe is near and dear to our hearts. They're nutritious, taste like an indulgent treat, and

leave you feeling satisfied and energized. See page 36 for more about this tasty temptation.

- Protein smoothie. For busy mornings a protein smoothie is Karena's quick-and-easy favorite. Toss a scoop of protein powder (like Perfect Fit, our specially made protein powder you can find at perfectfitprotein.com), almond milk, banana, kale, and some berries in a blender. Pour in a to-go cup and you're out the door in minutes.

- Mug Muffins. Mug muffins are Katrina's on-the-go favorite. Throw some egg whites with veggies into a microwave-safe mug, cover, and heat in the microwave for 60 to 90 seconds.

Don't worry, we're not forgetting the one must-have for some of your mornings: coffee! Just like you, we love our java (with a splash of almond milk). If you want to add a little sugar to your coffee or tea, go for it—in moderation, of course! A teaspoon of real sugar a day is 100 percent fine if it's natural (remember to steer clear of artificial sweeteners). We like raw turbinado sugar, but you can also use honey or maple syrup to sweeten things up.

Or get creative and combine your coffee and your morning meal to make our Healthy Coffee Milkshake! Simply combine the ingredients on page 37 in a blender and pulse until smooth and creamy.

Save Your Salad from Dressing Sabotage!

Many premade dressings can contain 400 or more calories per serving. That's the equivalent of running a 5-K! If you like to dress your salads, try one of our favorite low-calorie, flavor-packed recipes instead. Each recipe makes four to six servings.

Asian Soy Vinaigrette

We love this on chopped salads with chicken. Combine:

½ cup white rice vinegar

2 tablespoons sesame oil

1 tablespoon low-sodium soy sauce

1 teaspoon organic brown sugar (or 2 packets stevia for a lower-calorie option)

Balsamic Citrus Dressing

Great with chicken and avocado salads! Combine:

½ cup balsamic vinegar

2 tablespoons extra-virgin olive oil

½ fresh lemon, squeezed

½ fresh lime, squeezed

1 teaspoon sea salt

Lemon–Poppy Seed Dressing (keep refrigerated)

This dressing is great with chopped kale salads, in chicken wraps, or as a marinade. Combine:

¼ cup white rice vinegar

2 tablespoons extra-virgin olive oil

2 tablespoons plain Greek yogurt (0%)

1 tablespoon honey

1 fresh lemon, squeezed

2 teaspoons poppy seeds

1 teaspoon sea salt

2 packets stevia

Creamy Italian (keep refrigerated)

For those who crave something creamy, this will hit the spot. Combine:

1 cup plain Greek yogurt (0% to 1%)

3 tablespoons white rice vinegar

1 shallot, minced

2 packets stevia

1 teaspoon dried oregano

½ teaspoon dried basil

1 clove garlic, pressed

1 teaspoon sea salt

Dash of ground black pepper

your evening Daily Fitness Challenge. After you work out, your muscles are primed for absorbing nutrients, so give them what they need to get lean and strong!

Here are your do-good-for-you dinner guidelines:

Time it right. Eat dinner a few hours before heading to bed so that your body has plenty of time to digest and you can get a good night's rest.

Keep it real! Shop in Mother Nature's pantry and fill your plate with lean protein and fiber-fab foods (see tips #1, #2, and #3). Throughout the 28-day program, you'll find

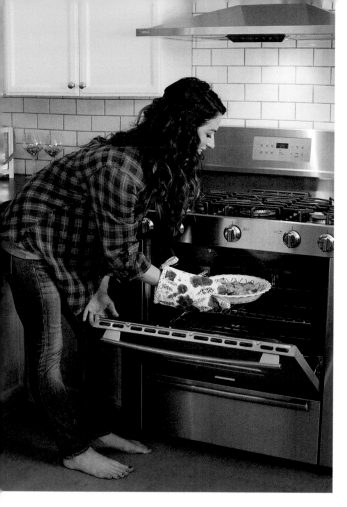

don't fret; you don't have to be an expert chef or have tons of free time to prepare delicious and nutritious meals. The recipes you'll find here and on our Web site will show you that it's easier (and quicker!) than you think.

Be a dining diva. Going out for dinner? It's your beautiful body you're taking care of, so don't be shy in asking for what you need. Ask your waiter to replace the cream-based dressings with something lighter and on the side (like oil and vinegar, so you can control how much you put on), or to sub out starches with veggies or greens. Request grilled fish or chicken instead of fried. Chances are they'll be happy to accommodate you—especially if you flash them that dazzling smile of yours!

Knockout Nutrition Tip #9:

Slow It Down

Why put in the effort to make or order delectable food, only to gobble it down without enjoying it? Eat slowly and savor your meals. If you usually eat on the go or in a hurry, it's time to change that habit. Gobbling down food means you're much less likely to register what or how much you're actually eating, mentally or physically. Worse, it leaves you unsatisfied, making you vulnerable to unwanted snacking later on. Plus, eating too fast can cause bloating, because you're not chewing your food well.

lots of delicious, healthy recipes to try, and there are many more at ToneItUp.com.

Get kitchen crafty. Fire up that stove, you gourmet goddess—cooking your own meals is your secret weapon for divine, waistline-whittling dinners! Besides being good for your wallet, cooking at home lets you control what ingredients are going into your body. Preparing a meal can become very therapeutic at the end of a long day, and cooking that brings together friends and family is a particular joy of ours! If cooking isn't quite your thing yet,

Snap a pic of your meals before you eat. It's a great way to keep yourself accountable and honest.

Meals are a special, sacred time to slow down and nourish your body and spirit. Linger. Savor. Pay attention and enjoy every bite . . . and the company you share it with. That, dear friends, is the essence of fine, fabulous dining.

Knockout Nutrition Tip #10:

Hydrate, Hydrate, Hydrate!

We can't stress this enough! Hydration is key in keeping your metabolism running on high and your body operating as a fierce fat-burning machine. Did you know that if you're chronically dehydrated (which up to 75 percent of us are), you can gain up to 10 pounds a year?! Your metabolism can't function properly if you're dehydrated; plus you're fatigued, so your muscles and joints can't withstand those fierce workouts you do.

In addition to keeping you hydrated, drinking water—especially between meals—ensures your body will tell you when it's *actually hungry*. A lot of time, fatigue can set in and we think we need more calories for fuel, but it's H_2O our bodies are clamoring for!

The minimum amount of water you need each day is half your body weight in ounces. So if you're 150 pounds, you should be drinking at least 75 ounces in water (a standard-size bottle of water from the store is 16 ounces, to give you a point of reference). Get yourself a personal water bottle and fill it before you leave the house. That way you know you have it on hand and will remember to refill it throughout the day.

If you're working out—and we know you are!—add 12 ounces for every half hour you sweat. The more you work out, the more you need to make sure you stay hydrated. And not just after your sweat session, but before and during as well. Being dehydrated during a workout can make it tough to get the most out of your efforts. Without proper hydration, your body can't cool itself down properly, which impedes your stamina and performance and can lead to muscle cramping. Worse, it can be dangerous. Throw a hot day in there and you run the risk of heat exhaustion or even heatstroke.

Along the lines of keeping it fabulous, you don't have to stick to just plain water! Lemon- and fruit-infused water are tops on our list of delightful drinks, and herbal tea, bubbly water, and coconut water all count toward your daily intake. We love to rehydrate with coconut water after a workout. We call it "Mother Nature's sports drink" because it has helpful electrolytes to replenish your body with the sodium you lose when you sweat. Coconut water also packs a lot of potassium, which prevents cramping and helps your muscles recover.

Water is your ultimate ticket to getting lean and light. So drink up, ladies!

Knockout Nutrition Tip #11:

Spice It Up to Slim Down

We love spices. From earthy and flavorful to kicky and hot, mixing it up in the kitchen makes everything more satisfying. Ranging from detoxifying to immunity boosting, spices are like the accessories of the food world. Sure, you can get by with the basics, but spices add that extra little something that makes the difference between bland and bodacious. So reach for the spice rack and embellish your meals with panache!

Here are just a few of our favorite spices:

Ginger. This zesty root beats bloat, aids digestion, and gives dishes a spicy little kick. Grate a little fresh ginger into your water or add it to your fresh juice or smoothie. We love

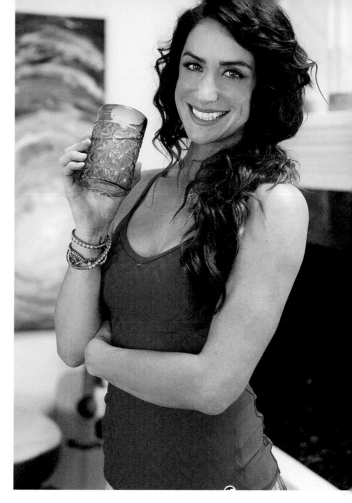

adding it to delicious recipes like ceviche, carrot soup, and stir-fry.

Cinnamon. Warming, comforting, and heavenly scented in healthy baked goods, cinnamon is a big favorite of ours, especially in the cooler months. It is a great fat burner and helps keep your blood sugar steady. Add a dash of ground cinnamon to your morning coffee grinds or smoothie, toss a stick into your herbal tea, or go to ToneItUp.com for plenty of recipes chock-full of cinnamony goodness.

Turmeric. Turmeric is the hidden

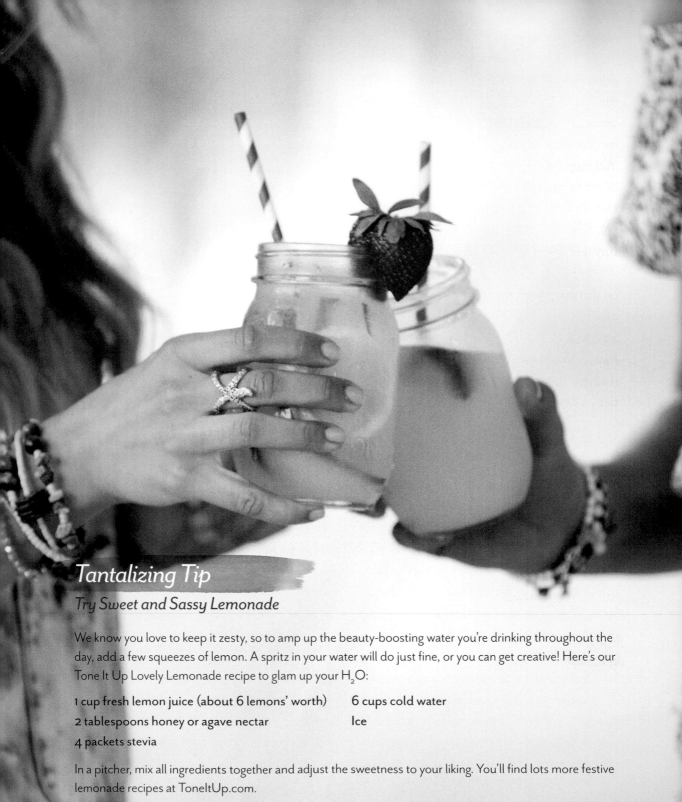

Tantalizing Tip

Try Sweet and Sassy Lemonade

We know you love to keep it zesty, so to amp up the beauty-boosting water you're drinking throughout the day, add a few squeezes of lemon. A spritz in your water will do just fine, or you can get creative! Here's our Tone It Up Lovely Lemonade recipe to glam up your H_2O:

1 cup fresh lemon juice (about 6 lemons' worth)   6 cups cold water

2 tablespoons honey or agave nectar   Ice

4 packets stevia

In a pitcher, mix all ingredients together and adjust the sweetness to your liking. You'll find lots more festive lemonade recipes at ToneItUp.com.

powerhouse in your spice rack. It has power-ful anti-inflammatory properties (great for workout recovery) as well as potent anti-oxidants (for smoother, more radiant skin). You might recognize it in its golden pow-dered form as the main ingredient in curry. Use it to add an earthy flavor to soups, chicken, scrambles, and veggies. For more on turmeric, see page 56.

Cayenne pepper. For a fiery kick, sprinkle on this sassy pepper. You'll hear a lot more about cayenne, which helps burn fat while adding zippy heat and flavor to all kinds of dishes, on Day 20 (page 146). For now, just know that there really isn't anything that doesn't taste better with a little cayenne sizzle!

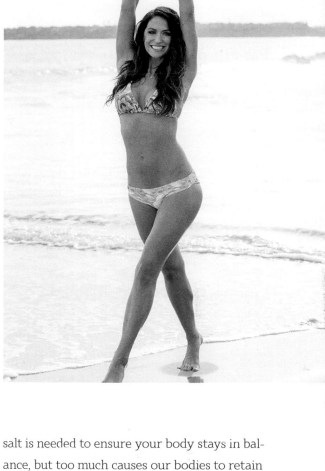

Knockout Nutrition Tip #12:

Ditch the Added Salt like a Bad Boyfriend

We've got just one word for you when it comes to salt intake, beauties: *bloat*.

Nothing can dim your shine quite like not being able to zip up those favorite jeans because you're bloated. A moderate amount of salt is needed to ensure your body stays in bal-ance, but too much causes our bodies to retain water, which blows up our bellies, puffs up our faces, and strains our hearts. Like a no-good dude, too much sodium is best kicked to the curb to ensure your well-being and fabulosity are preserved!

Many of the foods we eat contain sodium

I love a good kick to anything! I'll add cayenne to my morning egg whites and use it to season my lean protein at lunch and dinner.—Karena

Bye-Bye, Bloat

If you've had a particularly salty meal or just want a little extra slenderizing before you put on that bikini, here's your fast track to lovely and lean:

✳ Sip on peppermint or ginger tea. Both have been shown to get rid of bloat.

✳ Throw a piece of fresh ginger into your smoothie or fresh juice.

✳ Eat asparagus. It's been shown to be a natural diuretic that will help you shed excess water weight, stat! If it's grillin' time, throw some on the BBQ and enjoy.

✳ Add a squeeze of lemon to your water all day long.

✳ Drink, drink, drink water to flush out the sodium.

(especially restaurant food), so the trick is to avoid the excess. Do this by steering clear of high-sodium foods like soy sauce, ketchup and other condiments, store-bought salad dressings and marinades, canned soup, frozen dinners, processed deli meat, canned veggies (or opt for ones that explicitly say "no salt added"), pre-packaged foods, and even some cereals. The US recommended daily allowance is no more than 2,300 milligrams of sodium per day, but we like to stick to around 1,500 milligrams per day.

Knockout Nutrition Tip #13:

Treat Yourself

Let's get down to what some of you really want to know:

"Can I have sweets?"

Yes, of course you can! We love our sweets, and life is meant to enjoy the things you love. Just like anything else, it's all about moderation and choosing the right ones (are

I love a piece of dark chocolate. This decadent treat is rich in flavonoids and antioxidants too! Make sure you get 70% cacao or higher so you get the healthy benefits.—Karena

If I'm going to splurge, I love either dark chocolate with a glass of wine or a warm chocolate chip cookie. I always like to share dessert too, so the calories are half as much. And the moment is always that much sweeter when I share it with a friend.—Katrina

you seeing a pattern here?). There's a difference between indulging and treating yourself. The occasional dessert can actually help you stick to your healthy lifestyle. For some people, completely cutting out "forbidden foods" can lead to overindulgence later on.

We enjoy a bit of dessert a few times a week. The key is to choose high-quality options (you'll find many healthy dessert recipes throughout this book, as well as at ToneItUp.com) and start off by having just a few bites. You'll be surprised by how much less you need when the quality is good and you're really tuned in to each dreamy bite.

And don't forget about fabulous fruit for a sweet treat! Fresh fruit is loaded with antiaging antioxidants, essential vitamins, enzymes, and minerals. It keeps you young, fresh, and energized! It's also loaded with fiber and water to keep you hydrated and feeling full. Just to be ultra clear: By "fruit," we mean the real and raw stuff, not anything processed or "fruit flavored." Fruit in its natural form is so sweet and delicious—why would you ever want to compromise on its beautifying benefits?

Knockout Nutrition Tip #14:
Say Cheers with Confidence

Can you enjoy a cocktail in your Fit, Fierce, and Fabulous lifestyle? Absolutely! At the end of a long workweek, we love to get together with good friends and enjoy a cold bottle of sauvignon blanc while cooking dinner or watching the California sunset. Or, of course, pop a bottle of champagne if something calls for a celebration!

It's perfectly okay to enjoy a cocktail now and then—as long as you follow a few guidelines:

- Stick to no more than two cocktails a night, no more than 2 or 3 nights a week.

- Go with white wine, champagne, or clear liquors. Clear alcoholic beverages are lower in congeners, a substance made during the fermentation process that contains several chemicals your body doesn't like.

- Choose mixers with high-quality ingredients that don't contain added sugar. Say yes to fresh lemon, lime, mint, honey, sea salt, and other natural ingredients and no to premade mixers. You can find recipes for our favorite healthy cocktails at www. ToneItUp.com.

- Be sure to enjoy a healthy dinner beforehand. Alcohol on an empty stomach will make its way into your bloodstream much quicker. That'll set you up for a rotten night's sleep . . . not to mention a wicked headache in the morning.

- Drink water between each cocktail. Alcohol is dehydrating, so you need to up your

H_2O intake. Plus, drinking water in between cocktails wards off the dreaded hangover.

Knockout Nutrition Tip #15:
Do It for You

This last one is perhaps the most important nutrition tip of all, and it doesn't involve when you eat, how fast you eat, or even what you eat. Instead it has to do with how you think.

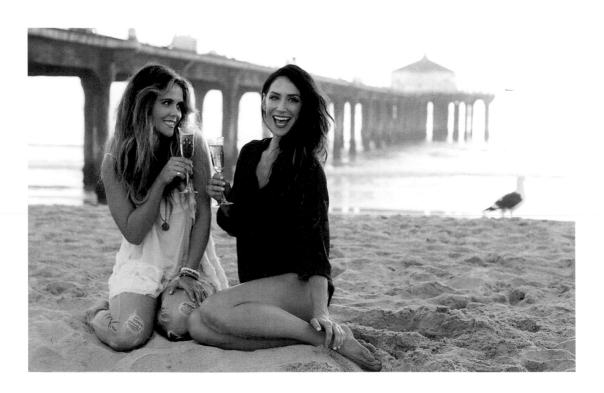

Tantalizing Tip
Give It a Spritz!

White wine spritzers are refreshing and delicious. They're made with half soda water and half wine, cutting the calories in half. Add a squeeze of lemon or lime if you like!

Fueling your body with fresh, nutritious food and forgoing the un-fab stuff is one of the most vital things you can do for your health and well-being, and we encourage you to see it as something loving that you are doing for yourself. Don't do it because we're telling you to—do it because it's for *you*! You are a fabulous babe who deserves a life filled with bounty and joy, and letting go of old habits to embrace healthy new ones is how you are empowering yourself on that path.

So eat nourishing, healthy foods because you *love* your body, not because you're forcing yourself. Do it for your glowing skin, your tight tummy, your sexy, shiny hair, and your loving, healthy heart. Let go of the chemicals, fake foods, and other fabulosity robbers and welcome in with an open heart the ideas you read about here. Experiment and have some fun! Choose delicious, inspired dishes that appeal to you and it will feel like a treat. No deprivation, no struggle, no misery. Those are what come of the "diets" you may have tried in days gone by, and you're done with those for good.

From our hearts to yours, we can promise you that if you live these guidelines for the next 28 days, you'll feel like a new woman. Your skin will glow and you'll light up every room you enter with your sexy shape, bright eyes, and sizzling energy. In other words, you'll be a *knockout*!

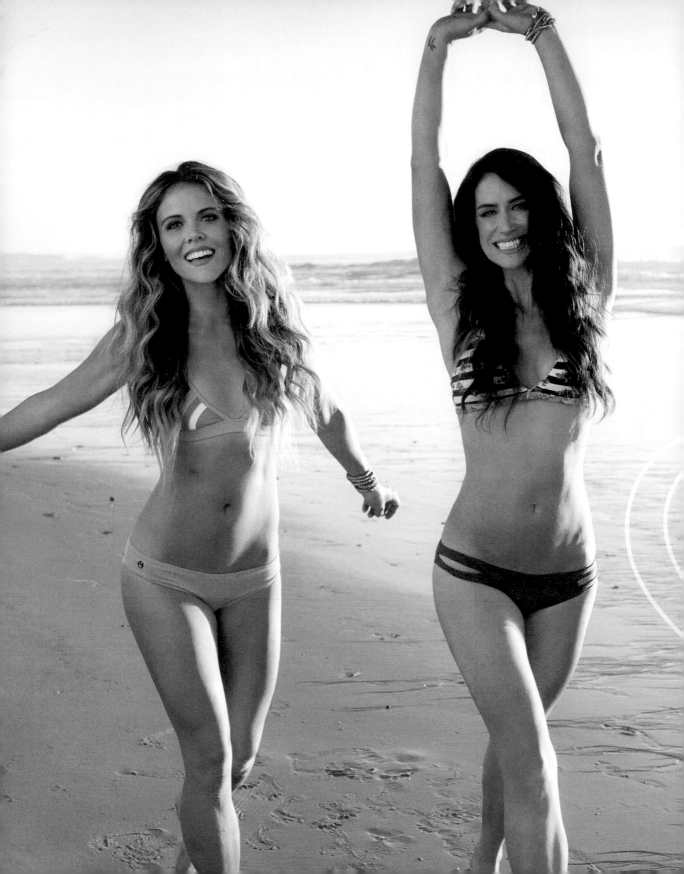

Part 4

Your 28-Day Fit, Fierce, and Fabulous Challenge

Ready to embark on 28 days of mind-blowing, booty-blasting, heart-opening, life-changing fun? Let's get to it, bombshell babes!

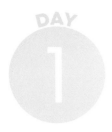

DAY

1

Monday

Your Word for Today: Confident
Your Mantra: I am strong. I am beautiful. I am capable.

Rise and shine, Sunshine! Today is the first day on your path to becoming your most fit, fierce, and fabulous self in every way. Yes, it really is possible, and yes, you can do this! You have within you everything it takes to accomplish your goals and dreams, and we're here to empower you every step of the way.

Maybe you're feeling a little afraid right now, perhaps worried that this will be too hard (you can rock this, we promise!) or that you won't be able to stick to it (you will). You might even be a little nervous about how your life may change once you reach your goals (no more hiding, no more holding back from going after your dreams!). Those doubts and fears may feel very real, but for today we're going to override them. That's right: *Ignore them!* Just toss 'em aside and get your strong, brilliant, ultra-capable self in gear, and very quickly you'll feel those doubts and fears disappear along with the pounds and inches.

> I don't think I ever really accomplished anything until I believed that I could. When I started to believe I could be the person I really wanted to be, it happened.—Katrina

All it takes is that first step, and your confidence will start to grow faster than you can imagine. We believe in you!

Be Fit

Here is your BE FIT plan for today:

* Morning Booty Call
* Daily Fitness Challenge: Full-Body Toning: Sweet-and-Spicy Strength Training (page 191)
* Fab Food of the Day: Goji berries
* Body-Loving Recipe of the Day: On-the-Goji Trail Mix

Morning Booty Call

We know, we know . . . the urge to hit the snooze button is super strong. But you're stronger! Here's your chance to prove to yourself that you mean business and that nothing will interfere with your rock-solid commitment to your new Fit, Fierce, and Fabulous lifestyle.

The first few days adjusting to a new routine may be the toughest, especially if you aren't used to getting up early. But the more you stick with it, the easier it will become. Pretty soon it'll feel like second nature. So silence the snooze button and wake up those lean, lovely muscles. You can do one of our Booty Call workouts in Part 5, or choose your own. Lace up those sneakers, roll out the yoga mat, or pop in that DVD. You're on your way, beautiful!

Fab Food of the Day
Goji Berries

These sweet little berries have superstar powers—just like you! Packed with antioxidants, amino acids, and vitamins, they are considered one of the most nutritionally dense foods on the planet (containing more vitamin C than any other fruit!). We love them tossed into a salad, as a topping for Perfect Fit Pancakes, or in today's On-the-Goji Trail Mix recipe.

Body-Loving Recipe of the Day
On-the-Goji Trail Mix

This satisfying snack is so easy to make and even easier to grab and go. Prep a few zipper-lock bags ahead of time and you're ready to take on the world!

Serves 2

* ¼ bar high-quality dark chocolate, broken into small pieces
* ¼ cup goji berries
* ½ cup raw almonds

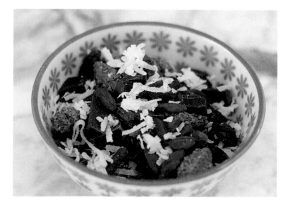

BOMBSHELL BONUS
Stretch It Out

Stretching after you work out is key to recovery, bringing down your heart rate and releasing any tension that may have built up. It improves your overall posture by lengthening those sexy, sleek muscles. Plus, it feels so darn good!

Plan a little extra time after your Daily Fitness Challenge to give your muscles a little love. Here are five of our favorite stretches:

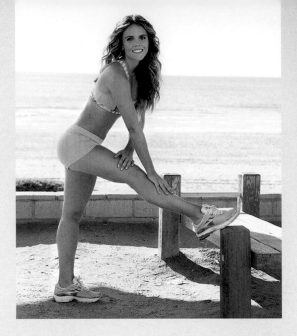

✳ **Calves:** Place your toe up against the nearest wall and your heel on the floor. Hold for 30 seconds and then switch legs (this hold time goes for all stretches, and always make sure to do both sides).

✳ **Hip flexors:** Start in a lunge position. Lower your back knee and lean forward until you feel a good stretch in the front of your hip. Want more? Reach back and grab your back foot for a deep quad stretch.

✳ **Lower back and hamstrings:** Sit on the floor with legs extended out in front of you. Gently round your back and fold your torso over your legs. Hold for 30 seconds.

✳ **Sides and triceps:** Reach one arm straight up and bend at the elbow until your hand reaches the middle of your upper back. Place your opposite hand on the bended elbow and gently bend your body to the opposite side.

✳ **Shoulders:** Extend one arm across your body and hold your elbow with the other hand. You'll feel this in the back of your shoulder.

• 2 tablespoons unsweetened shredded coconut

In a bowl, combine all ingredients and stir them up. Divide into two bags and enjoy when you need a delicious and filling snack!

Be Fierce

Nothing boosts confidence faster than keeping the promises we make to ourselves. Each and every time you follow through on your intentions, your belief in yourself grows until the day you finally get that you are a dynamo dame who can do *anything* she sets her mind to! That's the essence of confidence, and today you're going to skyrocket yours faster and easier than you can imagine.

Your BE FIERCE Challenge:
Commit and Conquer

At the beginning of your day, record in your journal three super-specific goals you are committing to accomplish today. Mental lists don't count—we need pen to paper (or fingers to keyboard) here. Writing it down puts it out there and makes it official—and that keeps you honest with yourself. These goals are different from the big, change-your-body-and-your-life ones you set for yourself before starting the program. We're talking about the daily to-dos here that usually start as good intentions in our minds but often drift away amidst the craziness of everyday life. (You know . . . like calling your mom or getting to that 7:30 a.m. yoga class.)

The trick here is that these goals have to be *tangible* and *measurable*. That means you have to be able to mark their completion in some way, and do it by a specific time. For instance, "I will be more active" is a great goal (and we applaud you for it), but how can you really measure if you were "more active"? Instead try something like "I will walk home from work tonight." That's specific—and it's something you can check off with an "I did it!" That's the difference between an intention and a goal.

Instead of "I will get organized," try something more targeted, like "Today I will sort through the pile of mail that has stacked up." Now that's a victory you can see! "I will be kind" is another fantastic goal, but let's make that real. How about "I will send my friend who is down in the dumps a special e-mail to brighten her day"?

Then, as you tackle each thing you committed to accomplishing today, cross it off your list. Actually physically do this, so you can visually mark your progress. Trust us, it will feel fabulous to see the goals vanish one by one. Ka-POW!

What will you accomplish today?

Be Fabulous

You were born to shine, baby! Today we're going to highlight all that's miraculous about you. No matter who you are, so many qualities make you amazing. Yes, YOU!

Now let's make that official. What better way to get that internal glow than to see all your fabulous qualities and attributes spelled out right in front of your eyes?

Your BE FABULOUS Challenge:
Make an "I'm Amazing!" List

Take out your Fit, Fierce, and Fabulous Journal and make a list of all the things that are spectacular and special about you. It may feel a little weird at first, but no one will see this but you, so don't hold back. This is no time to be shy! View yourself through the eyes of someone who loves you very much (ahem . . . you!) and write down everything that makes you the amazing creature you are. What do you like about yourself? Start with the physical, if that's easiest. Do you like the color of your eyes? The shape of your nose? Your graceful hands?

Now think bigger, to how you show up in the world. Are you generous? Funny? Wise? A loyal friend, a loving daughter, mother, or partner? Are you rock-steady in a crisis?

What are you good at? Do you have a flair for fashion? Are you a good listener, a terrific cook, a stealth backgammon player, a talented painter or singer? Are you handy with a hammer or skillful with a sewing needle?

What about all the things you do that make you so wonderful? Do you volunteer or show up for friends and family when they need your help? Do you keep your promises to others—and to yourself? Do you take good care of your health and well-being? Those all count!

Think big . . . or small. It doesn't matter. Your challenge for today is simply to come up with at least 10 things. As you move through the rest of this program, keep adding to that list and refer back to it whenever you need a little extra hit of that kick-ass confidence you're building!

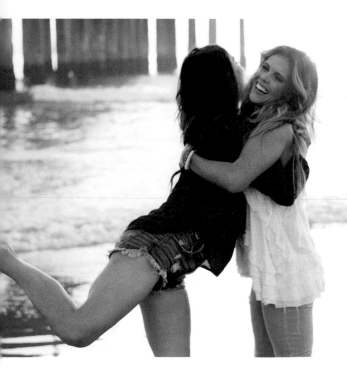

Name one thing that's special and amazing about you . . .

✳ I am a strong and dedicated person. When I put my mind to something, I do it.—Chelsea S.

✳ I am a loyal, trustworthy, great friend. —Whitney M.

✳ I'm a pirate! In high school I lived aboard a 168-foot tall ship and sailed from Africa to Canada with 50 other students.—Julia M.

✳ I have no shame about dancing in public. Like, seriously, none.—Katy L.

✳ My smile and my (loud) laugh!—Jenny N.

✳ I know a fabulous card trick that would absolutely amaze you.—Jillian M.

Tuesday

Your Word for Today: Motivated
Your Mantra: If I can dream it, I can do it!

You're focused. You're determined. It's Day 2, and you're well on your way, you feisty firecracker! Now let's keep that internal fire burning so that nothing gets in the way of you creating the beautiful body and life of your dreams.

Be Fit

Here is your BE FIT plan for today:

* Morning Booty Call

* Daily Fitness Challenge:
  Cardio: Go, Go, Goddess (page 242)

* Fab Food of the Day:
  Turmeric

* Body-Loving Recipe of the Day:
  Terrific Tofu Scramble

Morning Booty Call

How did your first Booty Call go yesterday? If it felt tough to get up and get going, remember: The more you do it, the easier it gets. You're going to learn to love it—we promise. Very soon you'll be bounding out of bed, *craving* that morning hit of energy!

Today is all about lighting it up, so why not try one of our HIIT Booty Call workouts in Part 5 to really spark your fuse this morning?

BOMBSHELL BONUS
Make a Power Playlist

Get yourself a kick-ass playlist to amp up your Daily Fitness Challenge! Sweating to your favorite songs makes workouts more enjoyable, and a recent study published in the *Journal of Sport and Exercise Physiology* shows it can boost your endurance by up to 15 percent.

Choose songs with a good, strong beat and lots of energy and arrange them to match the tempo of your Daily Fitness Challenge routine: a favorite song to start your warmup; more intense, fast-paced jams at the peak; and a more mellow set to cool down. At ToneItUp.com you'll find some of our favorites. We're happy to share . . . and don't forget to pass yours along to your #FitFierceFab sisters while you're at it!

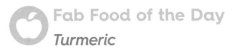

Fab Food of the Day
Turmeric

For extra support to keep you going strong, today we're featuring turmeric, which is legendary for boosting immunity. Its powerful anti-inflammatory properties are great for soothing sore muscles as well as increasing circulation and keeping your skin bright. We've definitely noticed a difference in our complexion since adding turmeric to our recipes! Sprinkle in this golden powder (or its liquid form) to add a rich, earthy flavor to veggies, chicken, scrambles, and more. If you can find the root, slice off a 1-inch piece and juice it along with other veggies or blend it into your smoothie to make it extra tasty.

Body-Loving Recipe of the Day
Terrific Tofu Scramble

We looove a good savory scramble in the morning! This turmeric-infused favorite is a healthy, easy way to power up and get your gorgeous glow going bright and early.

Serves 2

- 6–8 ounces firm tofu
- 2 tablespoons extra-virgin olive oil
- ¼ medium onion, chopped
- 1 clove garlic, minced
- 1 teaspoon tamari
- ½ teaspoon cumin powder

Tantalizing Tip
Like It Spicy?

Drizzle a little hot sauce on top for some sizzle! Our favorite sauces are the ones that use chile or habanero peppers.

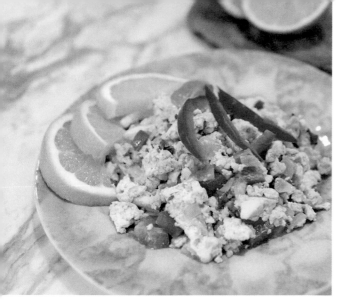

Be Fierce

Your goals are your ticket to motivation mojo, baby! They keep you focused, on track, and fired up. Making them happen is what today (well, really, every day) is for.

So what's the secret to turning your desires and dreams into reality? Visualizing the positive outcome you want to create. The key word there is *positive.* You'll notice we never talk about "banishing that muffin top" or "ditching those saddlebags." If you focus on things like that, then after you work out you're not feeling inspired—you're wondering if your saddlebags are gone. Instead we want you to focus on the strength you're creating within and for yourself.

Focus your thoughts and dreams on what you want in life and you will attract them. Yes, really! This is true for your health, your career, your relationships, and all aspects of your life. We have no doubt that you can alter your circumstances and happiness through positive visualization. Today you're going to gather up all your innermost desires and learn how to turn those delicious dreams into reality.

- Pinch of ground black pepper
- ¼ teaspoon turmeric powder
- 1 cup your choice of veggies (bell peppers, spinach, broccoli, kale, etc.)
- 2 tablespoons nutritional yeast

Press the tofu with paper towels to pat dry. Heat a pan on medium and add the oil. Once warm, add the onion and garlic to sauté. When the edges of the onion start to brown, crumble the tofu and add it to the pan. Lightly stir for 4 to 5 minutes, then add the tamari, cumin, pepper, and turmeric. Mix in the veggies and cook until the desired consistency is reached. Just before plating, sprinkle on the nutritional yeast.

Every morning I journal how I want the day ahead to go and set one specific goal for myself; most of the time, it happens exactly how I manifest!—Katrina

Your BE FIERCE Challenge:
Make a Vision Board

Ready to get a little crafty?

A vision board is a simple poster or bulletin board filled with a collage of images and words that represent all the good stuff you want in life. It can be anything your heart desires: a strong, healthy body; a love relationship; your dream job; or more. The sky's the limit, so dream big and invite it all in!

We like to fill our boards with empowering words and quotes that inspire healthy, happy living, like "Be present" or "You'll never regret a workout," along with images that inspire us, like a photo of a kick-ass female athlete that will encourage us to train harder. We'll also use pictures of things we want to manifest in our lives. This is something we've

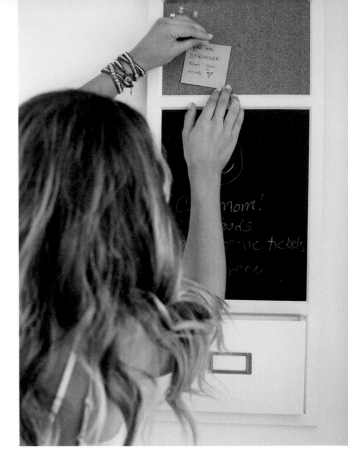

Of course we know that visualization isn't magic. It takes preparation and hard work to get the results you want, but I can personally say that having a vision board does help make your dreams real! Years ago, I made a board that had pictures of the Caribbean, where I'd always wanted to visit. Within 2 months I ended up getting booked for modeling jobs in Jamaica, the Bahamas, and Playa del Carmen. I also had a friend invite me to vacation at her parents' house in Cancun. I finally replaced those Caribbean pictures with ones of the French and Italian Riviera, and I just had the opportunity this past summer to travel there for work. Now I'm dreaming about what's next!—Karena

both done for years, so trust us when we say it really works!

Here's what you'll need to make your board:

- A large piece of poster board (or a bulletin board)
- Scissors
- Glue, tape, or thumbtacks
- Markers or paint
- Photos and clippings of things that inspire you
- A positive attitude!

Carve out a little time today and collect (or make) your inspiration pieces. You can draw the images yourself, tear photos from magazines, or find images online to print out. Once you've got a good collection, get out that glue/tape/thumbtacks and get it going! If you're more of a digital dame, Pinterest is a great alternative way to make a vision board. Either way, you don't have to complete the whole thing in one shot . . . just get it started, and you can continue to add to it each day.

Be sure to keep your board somewhere you can see it every day, to remind you of what you're reaching for and all the fabulous things headed your way. And please post photos of your inspiring creation at #FitFierceFab. The more you put your dreams and goals out there into the universe, the faster the results will find you!

Be Fabulous

It's time to multiply your marvelous mojo by connecting with another bombshell as fabulous as you!

Take it from us and the hundreds of

BOMBSHELL BONUS
See It to Believe It

Visualize your fitness goals—in detail—and you'll find yourself achieving them. If your goal is to run in the morning, but that snooze button wins every time, go to bed tonight picturing yourself lacing up your shoes, getting in that invigorating run, and coming home feeling on top of the world. If your goal is to feel confident in your body, imagine yourself rocking a killer pair of jeans and hitting the town with your girlfriends, feeling like a million bucks. Once you've seen yourself achieve your goals, they'll seem much more realistic. Create that mental picture and you can make anything happen!

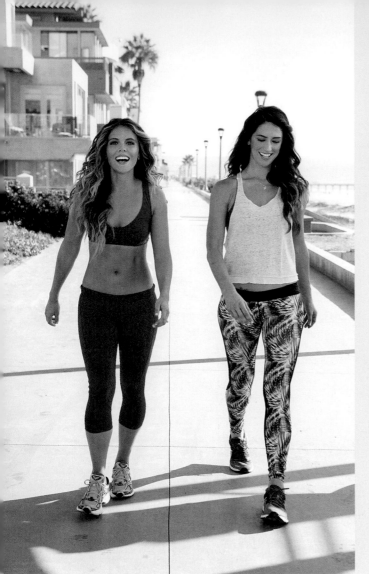

Who's your workout buddy?

✳ My friends and boyfriend always push me to try harder, and I love it!—Julia M.

✳ My workout buddy lives in Tennessee and I live in Connecticut, but we keep each other motivated via phone, text, social media, or by sending cards or little packages in the mail. —Jillian M.

✳ My daughter motivates me to push harder by having a healthy competitiveness. I try to keep up with her, and sometimes she tries to keep up with me!—Dina A.

✳ I have an accountability partner through social media who helps me get the workouts done on days that I'm not especially feeling it.—Stephanie F.

✳ My TIUpup is my workout buddy. He helps improve my workouts because he never wants our walks to end, so we always end up going longer than I anticipate.—Martha P.

✳ I have hundreds! The TIU community is with me every day, supporting and motivating me. They are the main reason I get my booty to the gym most of the time.—Candice M.

thousands of Tone It Up girls who never could have become the bodacious babes they are without each other: It's easier to rise to the challenges and get the most out of your accomplishments if you have a partner to cheer you on and keep you accountable.

There's something about sharing fitness and healthy living that forms deep and mean-

ingful bonds. We became best friends by sharing that passion, and we've also become accountability buddies when it comes to workouts and reaching our goals. We have a standing appointment every Monday and Wednesday morning that we confirm the night before. We meet at our favorite local organic coffee shop, grab espresso with a little almond milk, then take a short run over to yoga class. (We'll fess up: Sometimes we're a little late, so we have to run *to* the coffee place as well, because that caffeine is a must-have.) Some days one of us doesn't feel like going, but it's the other one's job to push the other.

We also check in with each other throughout the day with a quick call or text: "Hey, what are you doing for your workout today? Did you go for your run yet? What are you making for dinner?" Sometimes we even text pictures of our food if we made something really yummy, to inspire the other. As committed to being healthy and fit as we both are, we wouldn't have half the success we do without each other!

Your BE FABULOUS Challenge:
Find a Bombshell Buddy

Today make it your mission to find (and be!) a Bombshell Buddy. Whether you meet a friend every morning for your workout, have lunch-break walking sessions with a coworker, or even e-mail with your BFF across the country to check in on your progress, that support system will be a motivational miracle. You'll lift each other up when you need a boost, share tips, and create a happy, healthy lifestyle together!

Where can you find a Bombshell Buddy? The obvious answer may be right under your nose. Is there an acquaintance you met at a party who is into fitness? Someone you see on the same biking path every day or in your regular barre class? A coworker who works out at the same gym as you? Reach out to her and see if she might like to meet up for a workout (or even just coffee to start off). Chances are, she'll be so happy you did.

If you don't have an obvious partner in your area or in your contact list, a whole community of Tone It Up gals is waiting to connect and cheer you on. Go to the Fit, Fierce, and Fabulous section at ToneItUp.com, where you'll find thousands of women doing the program— many of whom are guaranteed to be taking on today's challenge to find a Bombshell Buddy, just like you!

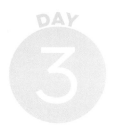

DAY

3

Wednesday

Your Word for Today: Centered
Your Mantra: I move through today with focus and poise.

We know you're here to sculpt a lean, strong physique and empower your mind, and we're right there with you on that. Very soon you'll have those, and more—if you don't already! But what drives all of that is something deeper and more elusive: the still sense of *you-ness* at your core. When you're moving and living from your center, it's easier to hear your innate wisdom and make healthy choices based on what's right for YOU.

Today is all about creating a reserve of inner peace and power. We'll show you how to keep your feet grounded so your soul can soar!

Be Fit

Here is your BE FIT plan for today:

* Morning Booty Call
* Daily Fitness Challenge: HIIT: Burn, Baby, Burn! (page 214)
* Fab Food of the Day: Beets
* Body-Loving Recipe of the Day: Sliced Beet and Arugula Salad

Morning Booty Call

This is an excellent day to focus on your core—in body *and* spirit. Consider rocking the Amazing Abs and Arms routine on page 247 or just throw a few power planks (page 233) into whatever workout you do. Feel the core strength building within and powering you through your day!

BOMBSHELL BONUS
Sit with Purpose and Poise

Most of us spend more than 10 hours a day sitting. YIKES! The way you sit can weaken your back muscles and, even worse, compromise the way your spine is shaped later in life. Plus, sitting all hunched over definitely doesn't reflect how fierce and fabulous you are. There's something to be said for rocking confident body language in the office.

All day, we want you to work on your core and posture. Focus on sitting up straight without collapsing against the back of your chair or rounding your shoulders. We like to set hourly reminders on our Outlook that say, "You are terrific. Now sit up tall and show it!"

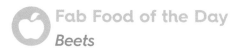 **Fab Food of the Day**
Beets

We've heard lots of yogis in our community say that consuming root veggies helps ground their mind and body. So this soul-warming, sweet-and-satisfying root vegetable is the ideal food for today! Beets are high in antioxidants and are a great source of folate, potassium, and iron. Plus, they add a beautiful splash of vibrant color to any plate. Who says that a healthy dish can't be fabulous, too? Connect to your roots with this yummy salad.

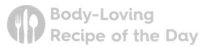 **Body-Loving Recipe of the Day**
Sliced Beet and Arugula Salad

Fresh, snappy, and bursting with flavor, this salad is just as beautiful as it is delicious. It's perfect as a side dish when you're entertaining—your guests will be dazzled!

Serves 2

- 2 large beetroots
- 2 tablespoons apple cider vinegar
- ¼ tablespoon ground cinnamon or 2 cinnamon sticks
- 1 fresh lemon, juiced
- 6 tablespoons extra-virgin olive oil
- Sea salt and ground black pepper, to taste
- 4 cups arugula
- Small handful sliced almonds, for garnish

Trim and peel the beetroot. In a medium saucepan filled with water, place the beetroot, vinegar, and cinnamon. Cover and let simmer for approximately 45 minutes, or until the beetroot can easily be pierced with a fork.

While the beetroot is cooking, in a small bowl, whisk together the lemon juice, oil, salt, and pepper. Set aside.

Once the beetroot is cooked, remove it from the water and slice it into ¼-inch pieces. Place the arugula in a bowl and top it with the beetroot. Whisk the dressing once more before drizzling it onto your salad and top with the almond slices.

Be Fierce

Establishing a morning ritual is a fantastic way to set yourself right before the craziness of everyday life hits. It can set the tone for the whole day and make a huge difference in how you handle challenges that inevitably come up. Having a few key things in place will help ensure you feel fabulous and energized throughout the big, exciting day that's out there waiting for you!

Here's what our morning rituals look like:

Katrina: I love to wake up and drink a full glass of water with a squeeze of fresh lemon while looking out at the ocean. It puts me at peace. I also love to go for a walk with my husband Brian a few mornings a week (Booty Call and time with my favorite guy all in one . . . heaven!). If we have some extra time, we grab a coffee and talk about our day ahead. Lately he's been making sure we leave for our walk before we open our laptops or phones.

Karena: Early morning before the sun rises is my favorite moment to make time for myself. I turn on ambient chill-out music on Pandora, light a candle, open the windows to let in the fresh morning air, make a hot cup of coffee, and just relax, give thanks, and meditate. I also like to use this time to read a few pages in whatever book I'm currently reading (while snuggling with my dog and cat!) and catch up on e-mails before I head out for my Morning Booty Call.

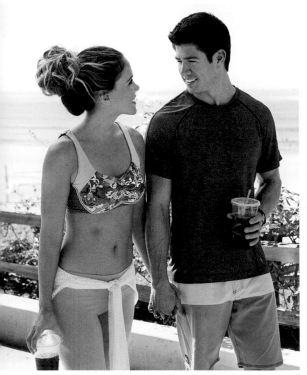

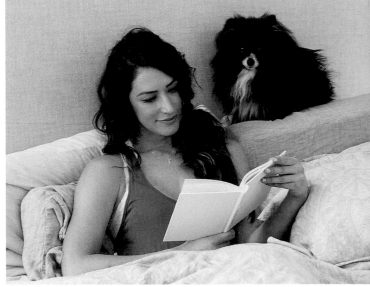

When I rush straight into my day and miss that time to center myself, nothing feels quite right. I need that time for myself . . . otherwise it's just 'up and at it.' There is such a thing as waking up on the wrong side of the bed!—Karena

Your BE FIERCE Challenge:
Make a Morning Ritual

This morning, set aside a little time for something that brings you joy. You're looking for the activity that makes you feel tranquil and grounded—even if only for those few precious minutes. Here are just a few ideas for you:

- Meditate (see page 66 for more on how).
- Sit quietly with a cup of coffee and look out the window.
- Read the newspaper or a few pages of a book.
- Write in your journal.
- Browse a Web site or blog you love.
- Organize your schedule and to-do list for the day.

Your morning ritual can be as long as you like and have time for, but try to take at least 5 minutes to get the most benefit. We know mornings are really busy for most of you, but 5 minutes are something everyone can afford. We all want to get as many quality zzz's as we can, so waking up at the last possible minute is tempting, but waking up just a few minutes early is so worth it. It will set a beautiful tone for the rest of your day. Do this for YOU—you deserve it!

You can do your morning ritual before your Booty Call if you want—we do! But after is great too. Experiment to see what feels best for you.

What's your morning ritual?

Be Fabulous

You've set your mind on track with your morning ritual . . . now let's add in a dose of sunshine to warm your heart and soul! Today you're going to get a little love from Mama Nature to get that healthy, peaceful glow on the inside and out.

There's something so soothing about the repetitive rhythm of waves on the sand, the trickle of a stream, or a gentle wind rustling the trees. Feeling a warm breeze against your skin or going for a walk in a winter wonderland of fresh, fluffy snow is almost guaranteed to relax you. Nature isn't worried about the past or the future. Nature just *is*, and being surrounded by and tuning in to it can awaken that sense of being present and patient within ourselves too.

Your BE FABULOUS Challenge:
Soak In Some Sunshine

This challenge is about as easy as it gets: Get your gorgeous self outside!

A lot of us end up spending all day indoors without even realizing it. We go from our homes to our offices and back home again, getting a minute or two of fresh air only when we walk to and from our cars. That's a surefire way to dim your shining light! So today we want you to take it outside. If you can, work out outdoors today. Hit a hiking trail. Take a swim in a lake. Walk in the park or on the beach. Whatever calls to you, make a concerted effort to spend some time under an open sky today.

BOMBSHELL BONUS
Meditate to Radiate

Meditation is a great tool for connecting to your inner self. It's a deliberate and conscious effort to recharge and refocus your mind. Not only is it grounding—it's also when some of our best ideas and realizations hit. And it's not just for yogis! Here are six easy steps to a simple meditation practice that anyone can do:

1. Find a quiet, comfortable place to sit. Don't think too much about it; just be sure you feel good in the space.
2. Set a timer for 5 minutes.
3. Close your eyes and take three deep breaths. Fill your belly with each breath, holding at the top of each for a count of 10 before exhaling slowly.
4. As your breath returns to normal, quietly observe the inhale and exhale. Nothing you need to do other than just feel the flow of air in and out. If any sensations come up, just let them wash over you. If you hear noises or feel restless, just let it be. If your mind wanders (which it will), gently and with love bring your attention back to your breath. Keep observing and feeling each inhale and exhale.
5. As you continue to breathe, bring awareness to your center. Feel the presence of your essence . . . your heart . . . your soul, and just be with it.
6. When the timer rings, turn it off and close your eyes once more. Take another three deep, cleansing breaths to end your meditation the same way you started it.

Stand up slowly and stretch for a moment. That wonderful feeling of calmness is now yours for the rest of your day.

Growing up, when things got intense for me, nature was where I escaped to. There was a river by my house, and just the sound of the water and the silence of the woods gave me a deep peace. Now it's the ocean that's my therapy.—Karena

Don't have time for a full-on nature workout, or weather not cooperating? That's okay; even a few minutes here and there can make a difference. Sometimes we'll find ourselves sitting in the Tone It Up office all day, and we just have to get up and go for a walk to rejuvenate ourselves. That 10-minute hit of fresh air clears our heads and energizes us. It's instant happiness, and it's available to you anytime you open your front door.

So get out there and take it in!

BOMBSHELL BONUS
Sport SPF, Rain or Shine

Make sure to apply sunscreen to all your exposed areas before you head outside (and don't forget your hands!). Remember that if you're going out to run for an hour, it means you'll be exposed to UV rays for that hour (yes, even through the clouds), and there's nothing fabulous about sizzled skin.

A good pair of sunglasses is also a must, to protect the delicate skin around your eyes. We all want youthful, beautiful skin and bright eyes for years to come! Look for an easy-to-wear, lightweight pair of shades with a frame large enough to cover the entire eye area. To keep them in place, we like ones that have a little bit of rubber on the nose and behind the ears. We of course *love* our line of Tone It Up Oakley sunglasses, which you can find at shoptoneitup.com.

I grew up going to summer camp—that's where I really found myself. Sitting on the rocks by the lake and writing letters home are some of my best memories. Years later, the sound of water hitting rocks still puts me at ease and connects me to my past and to my dreams for the future. Even the little tinkling water fountain in Karena's kitchen does it for me!—Katrina

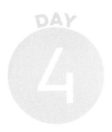

DAY

4

Thursday

Your Word for Today: Positive
Your Mantra: I choose to see the good in myself and everything around me.

Good morning, beautiful!

Today you're going to keep your mind-set moving in the right direction—toward all the good stuff going on, that is! You are in control of how you feel, because starting today, you're going to *choose your attitude.* Your happiness is up to you, and it all starts with jumping into your day with a positive outlook.

Be Fit

Here is your BE FIT plan for today:

* Morning Booty Call

* Daily Fitness Challenge: Full-Body Toning: Sweet-and-Spicy Strength Training (page 191)

* Fab Food of the Day: Lemon

* Body-Loving Recipe of the Day: Lemon-Garlic Stir-Fry

Your Morning Booty Call

What goes through your mind the minute you open your eyes? Do you grumble angrily at the clock and scan your mind for worries? Or do you smile at the thought of loving another fabulous day that's here to greet you? When that Booty Call alarm goes off, tune in right away to your thoughts and IMMEDIATELY think of at least one thing

BOMBSHELL BONUS
Roll Away Soreness

If you're feeling a little sore from your workouts—or just want an amazing way to release some tension—today is a great day to break out that foam roller. The benefits are incredible: It decreases inflammation, prevents injury, improves your range of motion and flexibility—not to mention that it feels great!

Here are the basics:

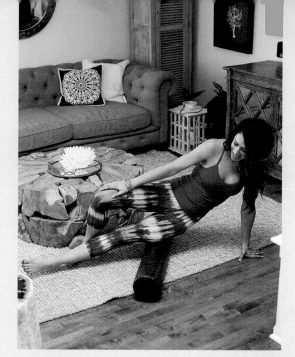

* Make sure your muscles are warmed up before foam rolling (after your workout is the perfect time to foam roll).
* Lay the specific muscle on top of the roller.
* Using only your body weight, gently and slowly roll along the length of the muscle, remembering to breathe slowly.
* When you come across a tender point, hold for a count of five, then resume rolling for a few sec-

onds. Repeat this process for 30 seconds or until the tender knot dissipates.

For easy, printable foam-rolling routines, go to ToneItUp.com.

you're looking forward to today. That's how we're going to launch your positive power today!

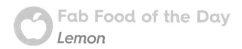 Fab Food of the Day
Lemon

When we think of *positive*, we automatically think of sunny lemon. This sassy little fruit helps detox your liver, combats bloating, keeps your body pH balanced, and makes you feel light, energized, and refreshed. Bonus: Studies show the scent of lemon makes you more alert and happy.

Keep squeezing that lovely lemon into your water throughout the day, and tonight cook up the delicious lemon-garlic stir-fry recipe on page 70 for a tangy, ultra-flavorful dish.

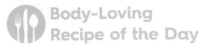

Body-Loving Recipe of the Day

Lemon-Garlic Stir-Fry

If you love Asian fusion, this is the dish for you! Skip the fancy restaurant or unhealthy takeout and make your own with this simple and spectacular stir-fry.

Serves 2

- 2 teaspoons extra-virgin coconut oil, divided
- 1 red or green bell pepper, diced
- 1 cup sliced mushrooms
- 1 bunch asparagus, trimmed into ½-inch sections
- 1 teaspoon freshly grated lemon zest
- Dash of sea salt
- 2 cloves garlic, minced
- 14 ounces extra-firm tofu, cut into 1-inch cubes
- 2 tablespoons fresh lemon juice
- 2 tablespoons chopped fresh parsley
- ½ cup low-sodium vegetable broth

In a nonstick pan, heat 1 teaspoon of the oil. Add the veggies, lemon zest, and salt and gently stir for 6 to 10 minutes, or until the veggies are cooked.

In a separate pan, use the remaining 1 teaspoon oil to sauté the garlic for approximately 30 seconds over medium-high heat. Drop in the cubed tofu and stir until firm around the edges. Remove from the heat and stir in the lemon juice and parsley. In a separate pan, sauté the veggies with the vegetable broth and a dash of sea salt and pepper for 3 to 5 minutes.

Serve the tofu over the sautéed veggies.

Be Fierce

You're training your body—but what about your mind? All your hard work won't get you where you want to go if you're negating it by being mean to yourself! Kat has a story we want to share with you about the importance of setting your mind in the right direction:

In my early days as a personal trainer, I was amazed by how harshly my female clients would speak about themselves. It made me so sad to see these beautiful, strong, healthy women focusing on and criticizing all the body parts they hated. Some would even grab a fistful of their stomach, bum, or thighs and express disgust. Who decided it was okay to treat ourselves that way?!

No matter what body part they complained about, I would always respond with, "You have such a beautiful _____. Let's just work and love it even more." I'd ask them to tell me at least one positive thing about their bodies. Over time, I saw their confidence grow as their focus moved away from what they hated to what they loved and appreciated about themselves.

BOMBSHELL BONUS
Enlist Your Bombshell Buddy

Negative chatter is a hard habit to break because it's so ingrained, so you have to gently keep redirecting yourself. This is a great time to ask for support from your Bombshell Buddy! Ping each other positive reminders throughout the day and make a pact to point out if you hear one another bitching and moaning—especially if it's about yourselves. One Tone It Up gal told us that when she hears her Bombshell Buddy tearing herself down, she responds with, "Hey, don't talk to my fierce, fabulous friend that way!"

Fast-forward to today . . . and to YOU. Today you're going to start loving that strong, beautiful body and your lovely life in all its amazingness.

Your BE FIERCE Challenge:
Nix the Negativity

Today we're declaring a complaint-free day. That means not saying anything negative about yourself, anyone else, or a situation in which you find yourself. No gossiping, no griping about traffic/work/the weather/your special someone—and most especially, no telling yourself that you should be better, thinner, smarter, or anything else. We want you to be the fiercest advocate for yourself, and that means no negative self-talk! As long as you're doing that inner name-calling thing, you're not going to get past it, no matter what you look like or achieve. Fabulosity on the outside only brings joy if you feel it on the inside too.

Kick those complaints to the curb for one full day and you'll be amazed by how quickly your outlook changes.

Be Fabulous

Positivity is contagious. The more you generate and share it, the more it comes back to you, and the more fabulous you'll feel!

Your BE FABULOUS Challenge:
Pass Along the Positive

Your mission: Give each person you are in contact with today a compliment. Yes, that's right—everyone! If the checkout gal at the supermarket is wearing a nametag with an interesting name, compliment her on it. If the person next to you in spin class motivated you to work harder, let her know. Tell a talented coworker you admire her smarts. There's at least one nice thing you can say about anyone you encounter, even if it's as simple as "I like your shoes."

While you're at it, don't forget your new girlfriends in the Tone It Up community. Check in at #FitFierceFab and let some of them know how much they inspire you. Chances are, they feel the exact same way about you!

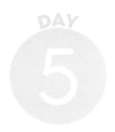

DAY

5

Friday

Your Word for Today: Gorgeous
Your Mantra: I am beautiful, inside and out.

Who, me? Gorgeous? Yes, YOU! You're a bombshell beauty . . . a magnificent mermaid . . .
a smokin' hottie, and we're here to make sure you know it.

Every woman is beautiful, and our individual beauty is what makes us unique. Trust us, we
all have our insecurities and things we want to change about our bodies, and we'll tackle this
more on Day 17 (Accepting). For today we just want you to take a leap and get on board the gorgeous express. It's time to embrace all that is beautiful about *you!*

Be Fit

Here is your BE FIT plan for today:

* Morning Booty Call

* Daily Fitness Challenge:
  Active rest day

* Fab Food of the Day: Avocado

* Body-Loving Recipe of the Day:
  Avocado-Cauliflower Spread

Your Morning Booty Call

Today is a rest day, so keep your Booty
Call loose and easy. Do some light stretching or
go for a slower-paced walk to allow your body
time to recover and rejuvenate itself.

You've been working your mind and body
like crazy, and now it's time to take a day to
slow it down. Rest is a vital part of this pro-

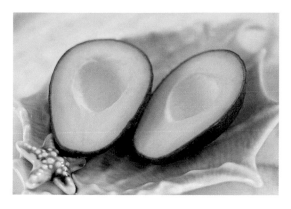

belly fat. Chock-full of vitamins D, K, and B$_6$ and essential fatty acids, it also does double duty keeping your hair shiny and your skin glowing.

Body-Loving Recipe of the Day
Avocado-Cauliflower Spread

Creamy and oh-so-satisfying, this pesto-style spread is perfect for just about anything! We love it as a salad topper or a simple dip for raw veggies.

Serves 2

- ¼ head cauliflower
- 2 tablespoons pine nuts
- ½ fresh lemon, juiced
- 2 teaspoons extra-virgin olive oil
- ½ ripe avocado
- 1 clove garlic, minced
- Dash of sea salt

In a food processor, puree all ingredients. Serve with raw vegetables or whole grain crackers.

gram; those sexy muscles of yours need a chance to repair from all your hard work! Plus, rest helps prevent injury from overuse and wards off mental fatigue. This is just what your mind and body need to keep going on your path to Fit, Fierce, and Fabulous.

Fab Food of the Day
Avocado

Avocado is one of the best-kept slimming secrets around. The healthy monounsaturated fats it contains reduce hunger and prevent blood sugar spikes that tell your body to store

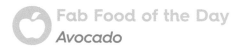

Tantalizing Tip
Tempt Your Eyes to Satisfy Your Taste Buds

Make your meals into a gorgeous vision! We're more inspired to eat healthfully—and more satisfied after we eat—when our food looks like a treat, so take the extra few minutes to fab it up. Use the good china if you've got it and use actual silverware instead of plastic. Arrange your food as if you were preparing it for someone special in your life—which of course you are!

Be Fierce

Now that you've declared a halt to the negative smack you've been talking about yourself, it's time to refill that pretty head of yours with the truth: You are glam, glowing, and GORGEOUS!

Your BE FIERCE Challenge:
Set Your Gorgeous Reminders

Who doesn't need (or love!) a reminder now and then of how beautiful and fantastic they are? So pull out some sticky notes and write at least three super-complimentary notes to yourself. Here are a few of our favorites:

- Hey there, gorgeous!

- Good morning, superstar!

- You are a glowing goddess.

- Your beauty glistens from within.

- You make me smile.

- Hey, hot stuff!

- Everything about you is beautiful.

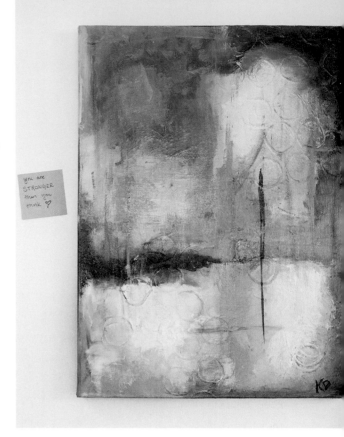

Stick these up wherever you'll see them throughout the day. Your bathroom mirror, the steering wheel of your car, and your computer monitor are all good examples. While you're at it, set a few gorgeous reminders to go off on your phone during the day today. These

We do this around the office too. Our staff writes and posts positive notes so we find these unexpected little gems of encouragement. I love how one sweet reminder can change someone's whole outlook. It's no wonder everyone in our office is so radiant!—Katrina

little positive pings can switch your mood instantly as you remember that you are truly gorgeous and blessed.

Be Fabulous

Gorgeous you deserves gorgeous skin and hair, and so today we're sharing two of our all-time favorite masks to send you into the weekend looking lovely and luminous through and through.

Your BE FABULOUS Challenge:
Get the Amazing Avocado Glow

Today's Fab Food of the Day is avocado, which—besides being packed with good fats to keep you satiated—is the ultimate natural moisturizer. This beauty bonanza is packed with vitamins C, K, and B$_6$, and the combo of these essential vitamins and fatty acids will keep your hair shiny and your skin just the way it's meant to be: soft and radiant!

It's Friday night, so settle in, get comfy, and take some time to freshen up those pretty locks and beautiful face.

For lustrous locks: Blend or mash together 1 banana, 1 ripe avocado, and 2 tea-spoons olive oil. Massage the mixture into your hair from roots to ends, covering every strand. Let set for 30 minutes, then rinse with apple cider vinegar and cool water for sexy, shiny hair.

For fresh, dewy skin: Blend or mash together $\frac{1}{2}$ ripe avocado, 1 tablespoon honey, and 1 teaspoon apple cider vinegar. Apply to your face and leave on for 15 minutes. Focus on your breathing and relax while letting it set. Rinse off with cool water and a damp washcloth.

BOMBSHELL BONUS
Get Your Gorgeous Groove On

Quick, name three things you love about your appearance. Don't hesitate—deep down, you know what they are. Do you have pretty eyes, a thousand-watt smile, fetching freckles, amazing arms? What do people compliment you on the most? Is it your killer curls, your radiant skin, your long, lush eyelashes? That's the gorgeousness we want you to focus on today! Remember, how you see yourself every day is what you become.

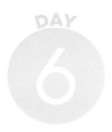

DAY

6

Saturday

Your Word for Today: Grateful
Your Mantra: I am so blessed.

On Day 4 you trained that sexy brain of yours to see the good in everything. Today we're going to shimmy that positive state of mind into your heart with the powerful practice of gratitude. We all have so much to be thankful for!

Be Fit

Here is your BE FIT plan for today:

* Morning Booty Call
* Daily Fitness Challenge:
  Cardio: Go, Go, Goddess (page 242)
* Fab Food of the Day: Black beans
* Body-Loving Recipe of the Day:
  Three-Bean Salad

Your Morning Booty Call

Before you get out of bed for your Booty Call today, place one hand over your heart and one on your belly. Give thanks for this healthy body you have been blessed with and for the ability to wake every morning with the motivation and tools to make each day your best.

Consider doing the Amazing Abs and Arms or Booty Short workout this morning to complement today's cardio Daily Fitness Challenge.

Fab Food of the Day
Black Beans

We've got much to appreciate about black beans! These legumes are stocked with two proven hunger zappers: protein and fiber. And thanks to their dark color, black beans are rich in flavonoids, to protect your skin from sun damage. But their beauty benefits don't stop there. As a bonus, the folic acid in the beans keeps hair strong and may even stop premature graying.

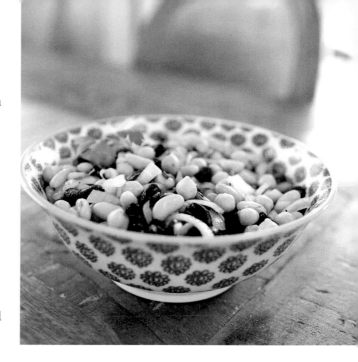

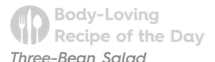 **Body-Loving Recipe of the Day**

Three-Bean Salad

This recipe is a fabulous favorite for picnics and potlucks!

Serves 2

- ½ cup organic no-salt added chickpeas, drained and rinsed
- ½ cup organic no-salt-added black beans, drained and rinsed
- ½ cup organic no-salt-added cannellini beans, drained and rinsed
- 1 stalk celery, diced
- ¼ red onion, diced
- ¼ cup chopped fresh parsley
- 1 tablespoon chopped fresh rosemary
- ¼ cup apple cider vinegar
- 1 tablespoon extra-virgin olive oil
- 1½ teaspoons honey
- ½ teaspoon sea salt
- ½ teaspoon ground black pepper

In a large bowl, mix together the beans, celery, onion, parsley, and rosemary. In a separate bowl, combine the vinegar, oil, honey, salt, and pepper. Add the dressing to the beans and toss. Chill in the refrigerator for a couple hours before serving to allow the beans to soak up the flavor of the dressing.

Be Fierce

It's easy to get caught up in the groove of everyday life and forget how truly blessed we all are. Taking the time to list the people you are grateful for and the gifts that surround you can significantly shift your whole life for the better. We're not talking about comparison or looking at those who are less fortunate than you. It's about looking within, at what you have and what you're thankful for.

Gratitude is the tried-and-true path to happiness. Here we'll prove it you. Right here,

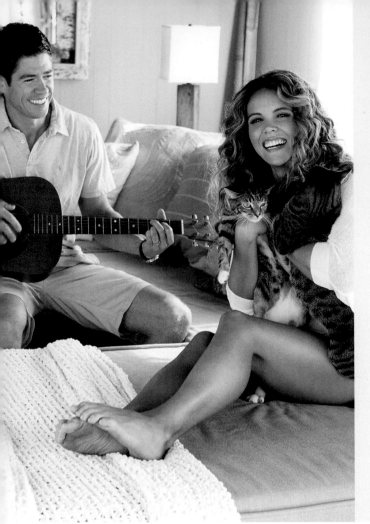

What are you grateful for?

✳ A body that works, each new day, my family (including the furry ones), my home, and finding Tone It Up.—Dina A.

✳ That I get to do work that I love—and actually get paid for it!—Ava G.

✳ I feel most grateful for my family. They have stayed by my side no matter what and have encouraged me to spread my wings while reminding me to stay grounded in my roots. I wouldn't be who I am without them. —Martha P.

✳ My girlfriends are risk takers, supporters, comedians, givers, lovers, fighters, den mothers, and all-around good people. I always feel so blessed to be in their company.—Katy L.

✳ Every day I feel grateful that the people I love are in good health.—Donna R.

✳ I have two of the sweetest kids on the planet, I'm head over heels in love with my hubby, and I'm so proud of where my life is going. —Kari B.

right now, think of one person or thing that you're grateful for. Pick something that is truly meaningful and precious to you—the love of your sweetie or family, your beloved pup or kitty, having a cozy home to call your own— whatever it is, really hold the image in your mind for a few seconds and let the gratitude wash over you.

Nice, right? That beautiful feeling right there, lovelies, is JOY!

Your BE FIERCE Challenge:
Take the Sunset Challenge

We like to offer to our Tone It Up members what we call a Sunset Challenge, to end their day on a happy note.

Here's how it works: Before you go to bed tonight, take out your Fit, Fierce, and Fabulous Journal and write down at least three things from your day that you are grateful for (more is even better!). Choose things that made you happy or just added a little twinkle to your day—big or small, it doesn't matter.

What happened from the time you woke up until now that's worth celebrating? Whatever makes you smile elevates you. Maybe you had a sweet chat with a good friend, got a flattering glance from a stranger, had a kick-ass workout, or just felt happy that it was sunny out today. Who in your life made you feel special? What places, people, or circumstances were you most grateful for?

Here's what our lists looked like today:

Katrina: Was inspired by a Tone It Up member's Twitter check-in to do an extra set of crunches this morning (OMG her 6-pack!!), shared an amazing piece of dark chocolate with sea salt with my BFF (Karena, of course! Some things are better when they're shared with someone you love), and ended the day with my favorite hot yoga class.

Karena: Started my day with a homemade latte and a yummy animal snuggle sesh, had a fantastically exciting meeting about new ideas for the Tone It Up community (I couldn't even keep my hands still. What can I say . . . I show my excitement through flailing body parts!), ended the day watching a gorgeous sunset with my love Bobby. And, of course, I'm ALWAYS grateful for Kat.

Gratitude has a magical effect. Besides elevating your mood, it holds incredible power to balance out—or even negate—the stressful stuff in life. Even if things didn't go your way today, you can always find at least a few things to be grateful for, and that brings things into perspective.

Don't just take our word for it. Try it and you'll see what we mean. It's impossible to feel grumpy and grateful at the same time!

Be Fabulous

As you already know, sharing the good stuff you've got going on inside magnifies it by a million. It's Saturday night, so tonight is great to spend a little time with a girlfriend who is extra special to you and let her know just how fabulous you think she is.

What do I appreciate most about Katrina? I know she would be there for me for absolutely anything. I love how loving and caring she is, and that when we have a conversation, she really listens. She supports and encourages me to take care of myself and live my dreams.—Karena

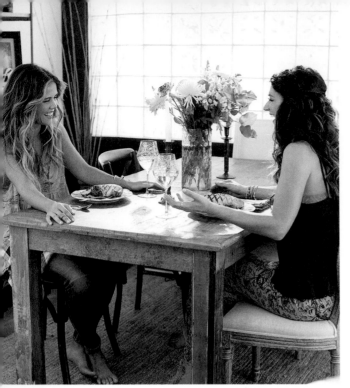

Make a date for tonight with a girlfriend you love. Set aside some uninterrupted time to catch up and make sure to tell her how special her friendship is to you. Even better, let her know EXACTLY what you appreciate most about her. If your best gal isn't close to you, make a phone or Skype date. Time with your girlfriends is priceless. You need your support system to shine as the fabulous star you are, and they are your lifeline. Chances are you'll inspire them to spill what they cherish about you, so it'll be a double whammy of love!

I love Karena's ability to make everything fun. She's always laughing. She never takes herself too seriously and can turn any situation into an adventure. I also really appreciate Karena's bravery. She's the most courageous person I know. I'm always the one that is afraid to take risks, but Karena encourages me to think big and leap. What are you most afraid of, but truly want to achieve? Now imagine Karena holding your hand and telling you 'You can do this . . . this is the right decision for you if you truly want it . . . you'll be okay. No regrets . . . GO FOR IT!' Something tells me you would do it. She has this inspirational power that is inexplicable.—Katrina

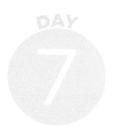

Sunday

Your Word for Today: Independent
Your Mantra: I am responsible for my own happiness.

Surrounding yourself with other Fit, Fierce, and Fabulous gals is phenomenally empowering and inspiring. But so is spending alone time with the one Fit, Fierce, and Fabulous chick who matters most: YOU! Get ready for a day of rediscovering your independence.

Be Fit

Here is your BE FIT plan for today:

* Morning Booty Call

* Daily Fitness Challenge:
  HIIT: Burn, Baby, Burn (page 214)

* Fab Food of the Day:
  Apples

* Body-Loving Recipe of the Day:
  Baked Chicken with Apples

Your Morning Booty Call

If you normally meet up with your Bombshell Buddy or others for your Morning Booty Call (or Daily Fitness Challenge), let them know that just for today you'll be taking a solo day. Tomorrow you can rejoin them, but we want you to experience one full day of just your own fabulous company.

Today is a great day to try the Walk Your Way to Wow Booty Call Workout on page 256.

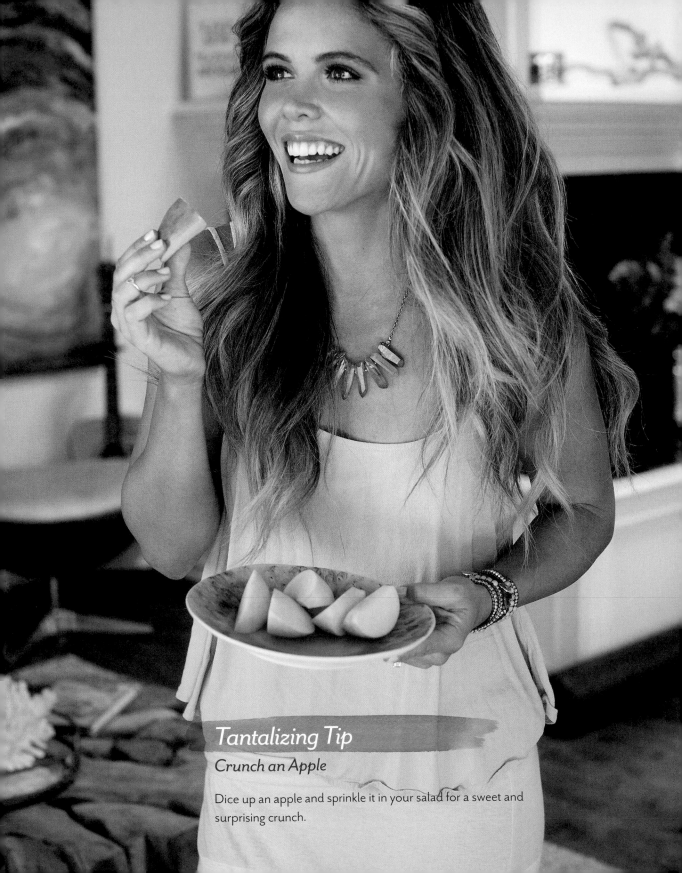

Tantalizing Tip

Crunch an Apple

Dice up an apple and sprinkle it in your salad for a sweet and surprising crunch.

There's something almost sacred about going for a long, lovely walk on your own in the morning hours.

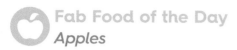

Fab Food of the Day
Apples

Need a portable, healthy snack to take with you on your solo day? An apple is the perfect choice! Sweet, crunchy, and packed with fiber, it stabilizes your blood sugar and will keep you feeling full throughout your adventure.

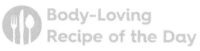

Body-Loving Recipe of the Day
Baked Chicken with Apples

Warm, filling, sweet, and satisfying . . . this delicious dinner is a can't-miss.

Serves 2

- 1 tablespoon extra-virgin olive oil, divided
- 2 boneless, skinless chicken breasts, 3 ounces each
- Sea salt and ground black pepper, to taste
- 2 teaspoons chopped fresh rosemary
- 2 teaspoons chopped fresh thyme
- 1 cooking apple, peeled and diced (good choices include Cortland, Fuji, Gala, and Granny Smith)
- $\frac{1}{2}$ medium sweet potato or parsnip, peeled and diced
- $\frac{1}{4}$ cup white wine
- 1 tablespoon Dijon mustard

Preheat the oven to 350°F.

Drizzle a baking dish with $\frac{1}{2}$ tablespoon of the oil and place the chicken breasts inside. Season the chicken with the salt, pepper, rosemary, and thyme, flipping it over to cover both sides. Cover with the apple and the sweet potato or parsnip.

In a separate bowl, mix together the wine, mustard, and remaining $\frac{1}{2}$ tablespoon oil and pour over the chicken. Bake for 40 to 45 minutes, or until the chicken is cooked through.

Be Fierce

Be independent and you can take on the world!

Enjoying alone time is important because ultimately only YOU can be responsible for your happiness. You have the power to make yourself feel safe and loved. Personal independence builds confidence—the type of confidence that will enable you to take the risks that lead to the fulfillment of your dreams. Traveling on your own—even for just a few hours—shows you that you can rely on your dependable self. Spending time alone can also ignite your creativity and lead to all kinds of amazing discoveries.

Your BE FIERCE Challenge:
Fly Solo

Go on an adventure by yourself today. Yes, that's right—just you, with all your confidence, smarts, and courage! This doesn't necessarily have to be

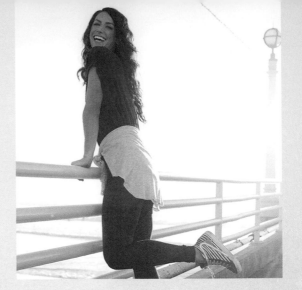

BOMBSHELL BONUS

Add to Your "I'm Amazing!" List

That solo journey you just embarked on took guts, so give yourself major points. Add "I am courageous" to your "I'm Amazing!" list from Day 1—because indeed, you are!

a major excursion or event. It can be absolutely anything, as long as you do it on your own.

Here are just a few suggestions to get the ideas flowing:

- See a movie by yourself (bonus: you can slip in after all the previews, because a single seat is usually easy to find).
- Go to a museum and explore on your own.
- Drive to a destination you've been wanting to check out. (While you're in the car,

crank up the tunes and sing out loud. No one's listening!)

- Have a solo shopping excursion.
- Take yourself out for a lovely lunch (bring a book or a magazine . . . no cheating and texting friends the whole time).
- Take a long walk and just wander.

So pack up your gear, program your map apps, and head on out there to discover how empowering self-reliance can be.

I love to cook dinner for one sometimes. I'll break out the good plates and sit down at the dining room table. I like to bake fresh salmon with herbs and veggies, or the flavorful kelp noodle recipe on page 88 that's my current obsession.—Karena

I like to do arts and crafts by myself. I made a lot of the favors for my wedding—I found that very therapeutic and fun. I painted all the little signs, made picture frames and collages, and then later made a scrapbook. I love to scrapbook! I grab a little time to myself to do it whenever I can.—Katrina

Your day of independence doesn't end quite yet. Tonight is all about YOU, beautiful! End your weekend with some fabulous beauty pampering and high-quality alone time.

Your BE FABULOUS Challenge:
Plan a "Me" Night

Cancel your plans. Turn off your cell phone. Tonight is reserved for you. Indulge a little! Pick something that feels like a luxurious treat. Give yourself a pedicure. Light a candle and take a bubble bath. Make yourself a special dessert (Tone It Up approved, of course!). Watch a chick flick in your pj's. Read a magazine cover to cover. The only rule is that it needs be a party of the one and only sensational you.

Enjoy!

What's your favorite me-time activity?

✻ Drink tea, take a bath, and binge-watch *Gilmore Girls* on Netflix.—Stephanie F.

✻ When I need alone time, I love to reach for a good book.—Chelsea S.

✻ I love to organize (accompanied by music ALWAYS). One of my favorite things is a clean and organized closet, drawer, basement, whatever . . . it lets me have my alone time and I feel accomplished when I'm done.—Kate R.

✻ A hike with my dog cures all.—Whitney M.

✻ I jam out to good tunes, journal, take a bath, meditate, or get outdoors.—Julia W.

✻ I like to find a coffee shop outside of town where I can be completely anonymous and sit with a warm drink and a book or a magazine, even if it's just for half an hour. —Jillian M.

✻ Go for a run.—Krystie S.

✻ When I need to reconnect with myself, I do a combination of looking up quotes, journaling, and unplugging from technology (especially my phone) to help clear my mind and refocus. I also find that I do a lot of my best thinking on walks.—Martha P.

✻ This may not sound like a big deal, but one thing I enjoy when I'm alone is to sit down and drink a cup of coffee . . . while it is hot! Having two toddlers at home, I usually end up reheating my coffee three or four times before drinking it.—Kari B.

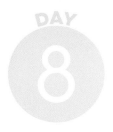

Monday

Your Word for Today: Daring
Your Mantra: I am bold. I am brave. I am up for anything!

We hope you're ready and raring to go after your rejuvenating weekend, because today is all about living BIG and BOLD. We want to hear all your tigresses ROARRR!

Be Fit

Here is your BE FIT plan for today:

* Take and record your measurements.
* Morning Booty Call
* Daily Fitness Challenge:
  Full-Body Toning: Magical Mermaid
  Moves (page 197)
* Fab Food of the Day: Sea veggies
* Body-Loving Recipe of the Day:
  Sexy Seaweed Salad

Take and Record Your Measurements

Pull out your tape measure this morning and repeat the same process you did before beginning the program, measuring your arms, waist, and booty (for a reminder of how, see page 18). The results will no doubt amaze you! Record them in your Fit, Fierce, and Fabulous Journal.

Your Morning Booty Call

Today marks 1 week since you've made the leap into your new Fit, Fierce, and Fabulous lifestyle—you're killin' it! You've com-

BOMBSHELL BONUS
Mix It Up

We all know that consistency is key to achieving a toned body. At the same time, if you consistently mix it up, you'll always keep your metabolism and muscles guessing along with keeping your mind and soul happy. So if you've stuck to the same Booty Call routine since beginning the program, today we want you to do something different.

Spice up your Booty Call today by stepping off the treadmill and hitting an outdoor trail instead. Or throw in some high-intensity intervals to really get your heart pumping (see page 221). Step outside your usual, even if just for one day. Remember, your word for today is *daring!*

mitted and put your intentions into action, which is a huge accomplishment. By now you're likely seeing some impressive visible results and feeling lighter and more energized, and that's fantastic. But there's so much more good stuff yet to come, so keep it going!

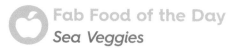
Fab Food of the Day
Sea Veggies

Venture someplace new to discover fabulous veggies: the deep blue sea! Kelp and seaweed are rich in essential minerals such as magnesium, potassium, iron, folate, and calcium. Think like a mermaid and add them to your salads or steamed veggies for a delicious, salty flavor.

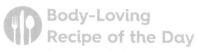
Body-Loving Recipe of the Day
Sexy Seaweed Salad

Intimidated by the idea of seaweed? Don't be! It's easier to find (and make) than you think. You can find good seaweed at most natural food stores and co-ops, usually in the Asian food section.

Serves 2

- 1 cup seaweed (wakame or your favorite!)
- 1 tablespoon tamari
- 1 tablespoon rice vinegar
- $\frac{1}{2}$ tablespoon sesame oil
- 1 clove garlic, minced
- 1 cup mixed greens of your choice
- 3 scallions, sliced
- 3 tablespoons shredded carrot
- 1 tablespoon sesame seeds

Soak the seaweed in cold water for 5 minutes. Drain and—if uncut—slice into $\frac{1}{2}$-inch-wide strips.

In a large bowl, whisk together the tamari, vinegar, oil, and garlic. Add the seaweed, greens, scallions, and carrot. Top with the sesame seeds.

Bonus Recipe

Miso-Infused Kelp Noodles

This, as you already know, is a major favorite of Karena's!

Serves 2

Noodles

- 1 cup kelp noodles
- 1 cup shredded carrots
- 1 cup thinly sliced bell pepper (red or yellow)
- 3 tablespoons finely diced green onion
- Sea salt and ground black pepper, to taste
- 2 tablespoons sesame seeds, for garnish

Dressing

- ½ cup light yellow miso
- ¼ cup water
- 1 tablespoon agave nectar
- 2 teaspoons tamari
- 1 teaspoon toasted sesame oil
- 1 clove garlic
- 1 teaspoon grated fresh ginger

In a pot, bring water to a boil and cook the kelp noodles for 5 to 10 minutes, until soft. Drain and pour into a large bowl. Add the carrots, bell pepper, green onion, salt, and black pepper.

In a blender or food processor, combine all dressing ingredients until smooth. Add the dressing to the noodles and mix thoroughly, tossing to make sure the dressing is evenly distributed.

Cover the bowl and set aside to allow the dressing to soak in for at least 15 minutes. Sprinkle with sesame seeds before serving. Serve warm or cold.

Be Fierce

Change is uncomfortable, we know. But that's the reason you're here in the first place. Branching out of our comfort zones expands our minds and lights up our hearts and souls. It is in the moments of discomfort that we feel something real and truly start living.

Fear is an indicator that we need to change . . . and change requires risk. Today, take it. No doubts, no holding back, no regrets.

Your BE FIERCE Challenge:
Do Something That Scares You

Today consider doing one thing you've always wanted to but perhaps were afraid to. Here are just a few ideas:

- Sign up for a 5-K (or a bike race, Tough Mudder, or triathlon). You'll be amazed by how focused you become when you have a deadline approaching. We always say the only difference between a dream and a goal is a deadline.

- Try a spin class.

- Talk to that cute guy you see every day in the elevator (bonus points if you ask him if he'd like to hang out sometime!).

- Apply for a job you've been dreaming about.

- Invite a potential new friend out for a drink.

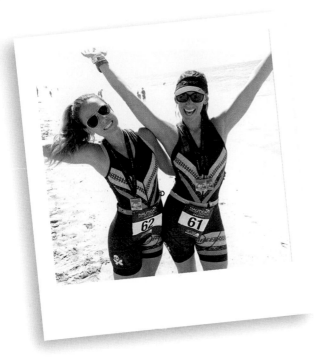

- Sign up for tango lessons.
- Do a high dive.

Being daring in one area of your life can give you the confidence you may need in another. So let nothing stop you today. Take action now. We DARE you!

Be Fabulous

We all get stuck in fashion ruts. It's just *soooo* easy to pull on the same colors (or lack of color) every day, because it's what we're used to. It's cozy and familiar. But when you shake things up in the wardrobe department and try something unexpected, it forces your mind to see things in new ways.

Ready to hit the fashion reset button?

When you reach into your closet today, choose something you don't normally go for. It can be something bright and patterned, dark and mysterious, or a creamy, dreamy neutral . . . whatever color appeals to you but you maybe passed over, thinking, "I can't/shouldn't/ wouldn't dare wear that." We're guessing you have at least one colorful piece hiding in your closet that you bought when you were feeling bold, but it hasn't seen the light of day. Today's the day to bring it on out and rock it!

Color has a powerful effect on how we feel, so pay attention to your energy throughout the day. You may be surprised by what you discover. Maybe a red shirt will make you feel extra empowered, or a sassy yellow scarf will give you a burst of positive energy.

Take a look at how colors can affect our mood and mind-set . . .

- **Orange** radiates warmth and happiness, promotes a positive outlook, inspires spontaneity and adventure, and represents independence. Its cheerful vibe expands creative thinking and helps open your mind to new possibilities.

- **Red** generates energy, determination, passion, and strength. This dynamic color is invigorating and packs a big punch. If you need a boost to power you through a busy day or some extra oomph to get through a tough workout, make this your go-to color. Even a splash on your nails or lips can do the trick!

- **Green** promotes healing, harmony, balance, and renewal. Think of how grounded and refreshed you feel after a walk in the park; that's the green all around you working its magic.

- **Blue** calms and soothes. It's a peaceful color that helps you feel mellow and mentally clear. If you're feeling stressed or overworked, something blue can simmer things down. Bonus: It also promotes a sense of trust and loyalty, so it's a great choice to wear to an interview.

- **Yellow** is the color of optimism. It uplifts your mood and promotes joy. This sunny color also enhances concentration, so it's a great choice to wear while studying or when working on an important project.

- **Purple** is feminine, romantic, and associated with confidence . . . making it the

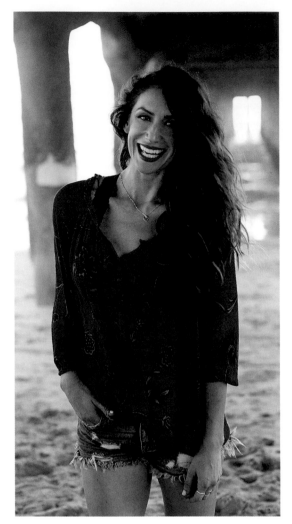

When I first met Kat, I was strictly a black-and-gray type of girl. Kat always rocks great neutrals with gorgeous pops of color, so she inspired me to mix it up. I started experimenting with new colors, and now I feel fierce and fantastic anytime I throw on something red or deep blue.—Karena

perfect color to rock on a date! It's also associated with deeper states of meditation and relaxation, so pull on the purple when you're craving a little soul-searching or emotional balance.

- **Pink** represents romance, compassion, affection, hope, nurturing, and sweetness. If you want to be in touch with your feminine side, wear pink.

- **Brown** is inviting and comforting. It creates a sense of practicality and simplicity as well as gives a grounded feeling of stability and support. Wearing brown can help you make decisions in a straightforward, down-to-earth, and uncomplicated way.

- **Black** is a strong, sophisticated, serious shade that helps you feel more powerful and in control . . . and it's also slimming!

- **White** promotes peace, calm, and clarity. Wear white whenever you need to clear your head or release negativity.

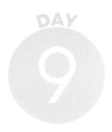

DAY

9

Tuesday

Your Word for Today: Connected
Your Mantra: I am surrounded by so many loving, supportive people.

So often we spend the day lost in our own world of thoughts and just going through the motions. Today we're going to pop that self-contained bubble and discover how inspiring and energizing it is to be connected and engaged with amazing people—even if we don't know them yet.

Be Fit

Here is your BE FIT plan for today:

* Morning Booty Call

* Daily Fitness Challenge:
  Cardio: Summertime Sizzle (page 243)

* Fab Food of the Day:
  Coconut

* Body-Loving Recipe of the Day:
  Chocolate-Coconut No-Bake Cookies

Your Morning Booty Call

Good morning! Open your eyes and before you do anything else this morning, go to the nearest window. Look outside. What do you see? There's an entire world of amazing people out there waiting to share in your fabulosity!

If you usually do your Booty Call on your own, today's the perfect day to try a group fitness class or invite your Bombshell Buddy to join you for a morning walk or yoga.

Fab Food of the Day
Coconut

We are c-c-c-*crazy* for coconut! Coconut water, coconut oil, dried coconut, fresh Thai baby coconuts . . . it doesn't matter. We love it all! Coconut meat and oil contains the healthy fats that are spectacular for your skin and overall health. We love to hydrate with coconut water, which is rich in potassium, and use coconut oil on our skin to make it soft and silky. Coconut oil is also one of the best oils to cook with because of its high smoke point (meaning it doesn't break down and get toxic at high temperatures). From smoothies to baked goods to a miraculous moisturizer, coconut is truly a delicious way to love your body!

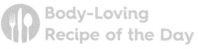

Body-Loving Recipe of the Day
Chocolate-Coconut No-Bake Cookies

Get your happy on and indulge your sweet tooth with these protein-packed, hassle-free treats.

Serves 2 (1 serving = 3 cookies)

- ½ teaspoon ground cinnamon
- ½ cup rolled oats
- ½ scoop or packet chocolate Perfect Fit protein powder
- ¼ cup unsweetened shredded coconut
- 2 tablespoons cacao powder
- 3 tablespoons honey
- 2 tablespoons virgin coconut oil, melted
- ½ teaspoon vanilla extract

In a medium bowl, mix together the cinnamon, oats, protein powder, coconut, and cacao. In a separate bowl, mix together the honey, oil, and vanilla extract. Combine the wet ingredients with the dry ingredients. Stir until fully incorporated.

With your hands, form into flattened cookies (5 or 6, depending on size) and place on a cookie sheet. Place the cookies in the freezer for at least 2 hours prior to serving.

Being happy is what it all comes down to . . . enjoying time with girlfriends and the important people in my life. Disconnecting from work and technology and connecting more with people keeps my heart lights on.—Katrina

Be Fierce

We all hide from time to time. Hey, we get it. Sometimes a girl just needs to hibernate to get her head on straight or rejuvenate. But when it becomes a daily habit, you're missing out on so much. The world is filled with caring, inspiring, supportive people who have so much to offer you. So let's go find them. Whaddaya say? We're with you all the way, right by your side.

Your BE FIERCE Challenge:
Look 'Em in the Eye

Throughout your day today, we challenge you to make eye contact with every person you encounter. Your eyes are the shining gates to your heart and soul. So look them in the eye and show them all the brilliant light that's within you!

Yes, that means making eye contact with people you don't know too. Don't avert your eyes when the barista hands you your coffee—look him or her squarely in the eye when you say thank-you. That gal you recognize at the gym but don't know? Look her way when she's passing by and give her your winning smile. You're almost guaranteed to have a brighter, happier day because of it—and so are they.

This is something we encourage you to do every day, but today especially, make this your mission and live your daily mantra.

Be Fabulous

How many times throughout the day do we miss out on opportunities to connect with other fabulous people? More often than you think! Today we're going to help you turn that around with a super-simple but stupendously life-changing challenge.

Your BE FABULOUS Challenge:
Say Yes

That's it. That's all you have to do: Say YES. Let in the opportunities and say yes to the offers to connect with others that come your way today, no matter how small they may be. If a

Take it from me, a former shy girl: When you aren't making eye contact or smiling because of shyness, you aren't coming across as the truly fabulous and loving person that you are. Others may interpret your body language wrongly and think of you as unkind or disinterested. So stand tall, look them in the eye, and flash them that beautiful smile!—Karena

BOMBSHELL BONUS
Join the Fab Fold

If you haven't already, today is the perfect day to go online and connect with other Fit, Fierce, and Fabulous gals who are doing the challenge (#FitFierceFab). In addition to your Bombshell Buddy, it's yet another support stream and source of ideas, inspiration, and motivation. You're not alone going through this challenge and change, and there's something uniquely special about doing it together with others.

coworker asks if you want them to bring you a cup of coffee from the break room, say yes. They're extending generosity and trying to make a connection with you—take it! You're not putting them out; they wouldn't have asked if they didn't want to do it (better yet, offer to go with him or her).

If a friend calls and suggests dinner one night next week, say yes. Even if you think you're too busy, make time for her and do it to keep that connection real and thriving. If your sister sends a text asking you to come over and watch that night's big awards show with her, go. Giggles and treasured memories-in-the-making await you. If an opportunity to join a group activity comes along, take it; you may be about to meet a kindred spirit. If your honey asks you to go for a walk after dinner, do it. Who knows what kind of magical talk the two of you might have along the way?

All day, pay attention to how often you're tempted to say no, thank you; give an excuse; or tell them you simply can't. And then each and every time, check that instinct to say no and do the opposite. No more rainchecks . . . today's the day you say YES! We promise, your entire world will open up in ways you can't even imagine yet.

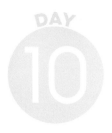

Wednesday

Your Word for Today: Creative
Your Mantra: I am an awe-inspiring ARTIST!

Every single one of us is an artist in her own way. Yes, even you! It doesn't matter if you can't draw, sing, or anything else that we typically think of as artistry. Art isn't about painting a masterpiece; it's about lighting things up with *your* unique creative spark. Today you're going to let your imagination run wild and unleash your creative genius. We can't wait to see what you dream up!

Be Fit

Here is your BE FIT plan for today:

* Morning Booty Call

* Daily Fitness Challenge:
  HIIT: Shred and Shine (page 221)

* Fab Food of the Day:
  Pomegranate

* Body-Loving Recipe of the Day:
  Baked Salmon with Pomegranate,
  Cilantro, and Quinoa

Your Morning Booty Call

Before or after your Booty Call this morning, take a few minutes to walk around your home and note what you see. Every single thing in there is a result of your artistry. The photos on the mantel? *You* made those memories. The clothes in your closet? *You* put those outfits together (okay, maybe with a little help from a fashionista friend or magazine, but still . . . you had an eye for how you want to present your fabulous self to the world). Last night's healthy leftovers in the fridge? *You* made those dishes (along with shaping your and your family's healthy eating habits). What else did you design in your surroundings? We're guessing a lot. You're pretty impressive!

Fab Food of the Day
Pomegranate

Pomegranates are associated with fertility and new beginnings (hmm . . . sounds a lot like creativity to us!). The vitamins in this sweet fruit have been shown to be great for your heart, skin, and immune system. Toss the gorgeous, ruby-red seeds in salads, yogurt, or smoothies or just enjoy them on their own for a snack.

Body-Loving Recipe of the Day
Baked Salmon with Pomegranate, Cilantro, and Quinoa

This classic dish is elegant enough for a special dinner party but easy enough for any night of the week.

Serves 2

- 1 cup quinoa
- 12 ounces wild-caught salmon
- 1 tablespoon extra-virgin olive oil
- 4 tablespoons chopped fresh cilantro, divided
- Sea salt and ground black pepper, to taste
- ¼ cup pomegranate seeds

Cook the quinoa according to package directions.

Meanwhile, preheat your oven's broiler on high. Line a baking dish with aluminum foil and coat it with nonstick cooking spray. Place the salmon fillets in the prepared dish with the skin down. Drizzle with the oil and add 1 tablespoon of the cilantro. Add a dash of salt and pepper. Broil for 5 minutes, then flip the salmon and broil for another 4 to 5 minutes, or until the fish is opaque.

Fluff the cooked, drained quinoa with a fork and gently fold in the pomegranate seeds and the remaining 3 tablespoons chopped cilantro. Serve with the salmon.

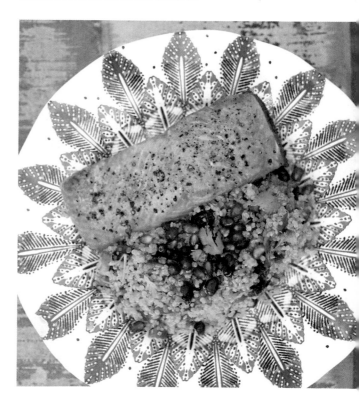

Be Fierce

Creative energy = passion. Passion is that feeling of being all lit up and excited, driven by inspiration and unstoppable in your vision. What could possibly be fiercer than *that*?!

Whether it's music, art, dancing, decorating, or anything else creative, everyone has an artist inside. It's a gift, and we're all meant to touch upon that in some way. Today you're going to find yours to become a PASSION POWERHOUSE!

Your BE FIERCE Challenge:
Awaken Your Inner Artist

Do you have an artistic streak that hasn't seen the light of day in ages? Painting, guitar, piano, writing, sewing? Whatever it is, set aside some time today to dive into it again. We both loved painting and drawing as kids and rediscovered that feeling when we picked up the paintbrushes a few years ago. Oh, that's a story you definitely need to hear! Here's how that all went down . . .

Karena: My mom is an artist. When I was growing up, our house was filled with art and her paintings. She inspired me to take art classes, and I used to paint big murals in my basement when I was a teenager. Life happened, and I got away from it for a long time.

A few years ago when I was back home, I did a painting with my stepmom Beth—I'd forgotten how much I loved doing that! I came back to California and told my boyfriend Bobby all about it, and of course Kat, because I knew she used to paint too. So one Thursday night, Bobby surprised us and took me, Kat, and Kat's husband Brian to an adult painting class. Picking up that paintbrush brought me right back to that free-spirited feeling I had as a kid. It was a time to get out of my own head and into a different part of my brain. This is such a fantastic mental release at the end of a busy day! Since then, I've made dozens of paintings that hang all around my house and in the Tone It Up office.

Sometimes Kat and I will have evening painting parties together. We'll open a bottle of wine, put on some music, and just start painting. Total bliss!

Katrina: I discovered painting when I was 8 years old and went to California to visit my grandmother. She painted for fun but was incredibly talented, and she gave me some supplies to paint while I was there. When my mom came to visit the studio, she was amazed by what I created, and she put me into art classes right away.

I painted for the next 10 years—mostly paintings for my friends as gifts (which is great when you don't have any money!). My high school art teachers were pushing me to study art in college, but I really just wanted to keep it as a hobby that I enjoyed and not turn it into something stressful. Making art is where I escaped from the drama of boyfriends and mean girls during those years. I was able to block out the world whenever I picked up a paintbrush.

When I got into exercise physiology, I stopped painting. Then I connected with Karena. She showed me the painting she made when she was home in Indiana, and that's when Bobby brought us to the painting place . . . and you know the rest of the story from there. Now I paint all the time, and it makes me so happy!

Karena and I use that same artistic ability in our work: photo shoots, graphic design, and writing our blog. Whether it's making a painting or creating our life together, we use that energy of creation.

Think you don't have a talent? We bet you do! Kat's husband Brian never knew he could paint until he took that class. Whatever sparks for you, try it. You never know. Intrigued every time you walk past a vegan bakery? You might have mad baking skills, but you'll never discover unless you try. Do you privately study how people walking by you wear their hair? You might be masterful with styling fabulous updos for you and your friends!

Remember, art comes in all forms. Bobby loves restoring old motorcycles; that's his art. Brian plays guitar and sings with the most melodic voice. You already know how much Kat loves to scrapbook. A friend of ours makes jewelry, and another collects interesting rocks and stones and arranges them in vintage glass

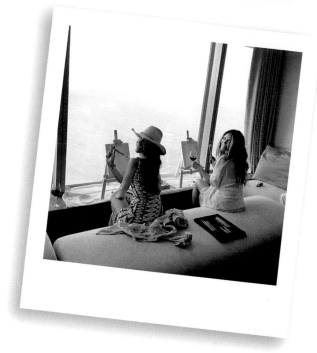

mason jars around her house. Art is everywhere; it's really just about finding the outlet where you're creating something new, given the materials you have.

You've already practiced being daring, so why not carry that energy forward and try something artistic that scares you a little? Sign up for a pottery-making or African drumming class. Go into your local knitting store and ask them to show you the basics. Do karaoke. Whatever you've secretly always wanted to try, today's the day to go for it!

Be Fabulous

Ultimately art is all about creating pockets of beauty in your life. You can be a master at so many things that enhance the gorgeous goddess you are. Makeup, clothes, hairstyles: It's all art.

Your BE FABULOUS Challenge: Have Some Fun with Your Closet

How many times have you been running late to a date night or when meeting up with girlfriends because you have "nothing to wear"? Time to fix that—and without spending a penny! With just a little creativity, unhurried time, and a sense of adventure, you'll be astonished by what you can create from what's already in your closet.

Today have some fun and play dress up. We challenge you to put together five fun looks based on the pieces you already own. Be daring and mix different colors or patterns you normally wouldn't. Be sure to accessorize too! Snap a quick pic of each outfit and keep them on your phone for a quick reference.

For an extra hit of fun, invite a girlfriend over to help and get a fresh set of eyes on your wardrobe. Make a party out of it!

How do you get your creative groove on?

✱ I love to write and only recently got back into it thanks to a push from my great TIU friend. —Amy M.

✱ My mom and I get together around the holidays and make wreaths. We play Christmas music and laugh and I just cherish that time so much.—Tiffany M.

✱ Cooking! I love to make up recipes.—Julia W.

✱ Putting together outfits I feel confident in and that reflect my personal style.—Jillian M.

✱ I love making things for my apartment decor, gifts for loved ones, or something as simple as a handmade card.—Erica H.

✱ I can (and will) dance to anything, anywhere, anytime.—Katy L.

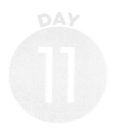

DAY

11

Thursday

Your Word for Today: Empowered
Your Mantra: Taking care of myself matters, both for me and for others.

Your word for today is *empowered*, which means "having been given authority." And you know who has the authority over you and your life, don't you? That's right, you righteous babe: YOU! So take on today with the intention of giving yourself permission to take care of your needs and be in charge of your own destiny.

Be Fit

Here is your BE FIT plan for today:

* Morning Booty Call

* Daily Fitness Challenge:
  Full-Body Toning: Magical Mermaid
  Moves (page 197)

* Fab Food of the Day:
  Leafy greens

* Body-Loving Recipe of the Day:
  Komforting Kale

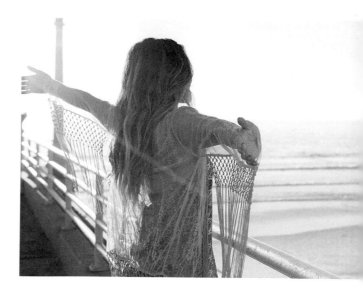

Your Morning Booty Call

Welcome to Thrivin' Thursday! What do you most need this morning to feel at your best? Is it your morning ritual, a revved-up Booty Call, an extra-long hot shower? Today is all about taking care of you, so tune in to what is essential for your well-being.

Fab Food of the Day
Leafy Greens

From kick-ass kale to awesome arugula, leafy greens are nutrient POWERBOMBS. They make your body beautiful, inside and out. Raw greens contain more minerals and enzymes than almost any other food. They alkalize your body, cleanse your digestive system, and fuel your workouts by keeping you healthy and energized. Nourish your sexy body every day with dark, leafy greens and watch it transform!

Body-Loving Recipe of the Day
Komforting Kale

You can never have too many great kale recipes! This one is a warm, comforting take on the traditional with a hint of garlic and red pepper to spice things up.

Serves 2

- 2 tablespoons extra-virgin olive oil
- 1 clove garlic, minced
- ½ cup cherry tomatoes, halved
- 2 bunches kale, chopped (with stems removed), divided
- 2 tablespoons pine nuts
- ½ teaspoon red pepper flakes
- Sea salt and ground black pepper, to taste

In a large pan on low heat, heat the oil. Add the garlic and cherry tomatoes and stir for 2 minutes. Add 1 bunch of kale leaves and cook for 1 to 2 minutes. Add the second bunch of kale and continue to sauté for about 3 minutes longer. Toss in the pine nuts, red pepper flakes, salt, and pepper and stir. Continue cooking until the kale is tender but still bright green.

Be Fierce

Just like you, we're usually super busy working, traveling, working some more, and taking care of the people we love. We 100 percent understand what it's like to be on the go and wanting to show up for everything and everyone who is important to you. And still, we also know how important it is to take the time to focus on our own needs. For many of us, that's not our natural instinct. But sometimes it needs to be.

Like today, for instance!

Your BE FIERCE Challenge:
Put YOU First

Today we want you to build your nonnegotiable list for putting yourself first. This is a daily checklist of the things you absolutely, positively should not and will not neglect.

Here's what ours look like:

Katrina's Daily Nonnegotiables

- Workout! This needs to happen for me to be happy in mind, body, and soul
- Writing in my journal
- Preparing healthy meals for myself
- Making my space special. Whether I'm at the office or at home, I am at my best when I make a happy environment for myself with fresh flowers, a comfy seat, pictures of people and places I love, and soothing music.

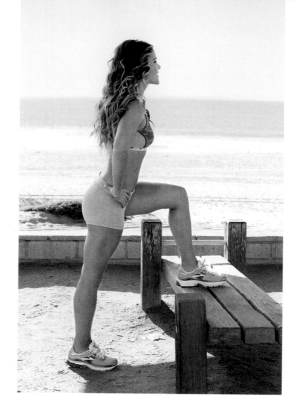

BOMBSHELL BONUS
Say Good-Bye to Guilt

Letting go of guilt is a huge step to becoming the FIERCE babe you are! As women we hold a lot of responsibility to take care of our home, have a career, and make sure our significant other and children are happy and taken care of. We often feel guilty for spending any time on ourselves or doing something we love. But really, that's just more negative self-talk, and you're already well on your way to kicking that habit to the curb.

When you feel that tug at your heart, you just have to talk yourself through it. First figure out what it is. Do you have a right you need to wrong? If there's something real that's amiss, is there one thing you can do that would enable you to let that go? Send an e-mail, make a date for another time, whatever it is . . . do it and move on! Or are you just feeling guilty because that's your default? Spend some time and dig deep to see why you're feeling that way. You may find you're holding on to a fear of abandonment or other insecurities from the past or taking on a victim role. Whatever it is that's gnawing at you, release it. You're appreciated and loved exactly as you are today.

• No cell phone for an hour before bed. That's my time to disconnect from the world, reflect on the day, and reconnect with my husband.

Karena's Daily Nonnegotiables

• Morning time with myself to set my intentions and goals for the day

• At least one sweat session

• Whatever beauty ritual I need that day, whether it's getting a manicure, doing a hair mask, taking a steam shower, or getting a massage. I need one thing that makes me feel good, inside and out!

What matters most to you? What do you need on a daily basis to feel centered, calm, happy—and empowered?

Be Fabulous

A bold, fresh lip color will make you feel unstoppable! Whether you have a drawer full of lip color to choose from or decide to treat yourself to something new, today's a day to find your favorite shade and rock it all day long: at work, school, even at the gym. Your bright, shiny lips will make you feel confident and beautiful—just like the knockout you are!

What are your daily nonnegotiables?

✳ My workouts, spend time with my boyfriend and dogs, a nice shower.—Krystie S.

✳ Yoga. Pray. Coffee.—Stephanie F.

✳ Check in with the TIU community online, eat healthy, and work out.—Julia M.

✳ Prep/pack a healthy breakfast and lunch. Food is such a central part of my life, not only for fuel, but for enjoyment! When I can make something healthy and delicious for myself, I feel so happy and accomplished.—Kate R.

✳ Each day I have to go for a run, and I have to have to have to have coffee! I also make sure no matter how hectic the workday gets, I try and get away from my desk for at least 15 minutes and go for a walk.—Tiffany M.

✳ Breathe. Kiss my fiancé. And most importantly, sleep well.—Whitney M.

✳ Express gratitude, group chat my friends and family, and drink all my water!—Julia M.

✳ Talk with my mom and sister, spend quality time with my TIUpup, and prep for the next day as soon as I get home so I can have the rest of the evening available.—Martha P.

✳ Have a satisfying breakfast (sets me up for the whole day) and laugh really, really loud. —Katy L.

I know I carry a lot of guilt about not being a good friend when I'm distracted with work, or even just want to be by myself. But I've learned that it's okay to dedicate time to myself, because that makes me the fierce and fabulous friend they actually want to be around.—Karena

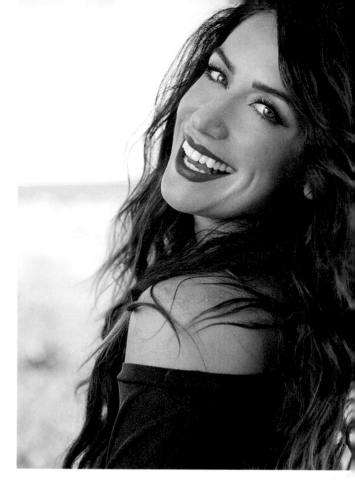

Your BE FABULOUS Challenge:
Pack a Lip-Smacking Punch

Try our tips for a world-class kisser:

- Nothing says "kiss me" like soft, silky lips, so keep your smackaroos supple with an SPF lip balm—all the better if it smells delish (try our coconut or pineapple Bombshell Balm to transport you to your own tropical island).

- Rock a killer red for major oomph. Studies from the *Journal of Social Psychology* show that the color red amps up attractiveness. Red lips have been proven to increase the sexy factor and give off an "I'm-so-hot-right-now" aura! (Bonus tip: Our favorite way to show off bright lips is to stick to natural makeup. Add a little bronzer, nude eye shadow, and mascara, and BAM . . . you're irresistible!)

- Go subtle and sassy with a sheer coral lip. This is Kat's obsession! It's a little sweet, a little bold, and totally bombshell babe-alicious.

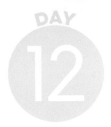

DAY

12

Friday

Your Word for Today: Reflective
Your Mantra: All I need to know comes from within.

Today you'll do a little check-in with yourself to get a reading on where you are in body and mind as well as what's come up for you in the program so far. Breathe, review, reflect: Those are your quiet but meaningful goals for today.

Be Fit

Here is your BE FIT plan for today:

* Morning Booty Call

* Daily Fitness Challenge:
  Cardio: Summertime Sizzle (page 243)

* Fab Food of the Day: Hemp seeds

* Body-Loving Recipe of the Day:
  Hemp Seed Salad

Your Morning Booty Call

How are your Booty Calls going so far? Today we want you to check in with yourself about your sunrise sessions. What's worked best for you? What did you enjoy most? What was challenging? Take an inventory of what's worked, what hasn't, and what you want to try next.

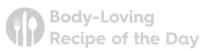 Fab Food of the Day
Hemp Seeds

Protein-packed hemp seeds deliver tons of nutrients along with their appealing nutty flavor. Sprinkle them into soups and salads for muscle repair and workout recovery, and for lustrous skin, hair, and nails.

Body-Loving Recipe of the Day
Hemp Seed Salad

A green, hearty, nutty, and lip-smackingly good salad with the creamiest, dreamiest dressing you've ever tried!

Serves 2

Salad

- ½ cucumber, diced
- 2 cups fresh spinach
- 1 cup diced fresh tomatoes
- 1 can (15 ounces) white beans, drained and rinsed
- 1 cup organic corn kernels (canned, no sodium added)
- 1 green bell pepper, diced
- 3 tablespoons hemp seeds

Heavenly Hemp Dressing

- ½ avocado, mashed
- 1 fresh lemon, juiced
- ¼ teaspoon sea salt
- 1 tablespoon hemp seeds
- ¼ teaspoon garlic powder

In a large bowl, combine all salad ingredients. In a separate bowl, whisk together the dressing ingredients until smooth. Pour the dressing over the salad mixture and stir. Refrigerate for 20 minutes before serving.

Be Fierce

As you travel through your day, tune in and pay attention to what you're thinking and how you're feeling. The more you can get in touch with your innermost thoughts and emotions, the more powerful you become, because you are able to see ahead to the obstacles and plan best for your successes. This is all part of building your inner fierceness as you get to know the wisdom of your own mind and heart.

Your BE FIERCE Challenge:
Rewind to Move Forward

Take out your journal when you have some unhurried alone time today. Open to a fresh page and spend a little time journaling your answers to these questions about your Fit, Fierce, and Fabulous experience thus far:

- How do I feel in my body today?
- What improvements have I seen in how I look and feel?
- What is most on my mind today? What am I feeling?

- How has the way I think and feel about myself changed since Day 1?
- Which of the BE FIT, BE FIERCE, and BE FABULOUS challenges did I like the most?
- What are my biggest triumphs so far on this program?
- What was most challenging for me?
- How did I overcome that challenge—or what can I put in place to help me with that?
- What do I most want to happen next?

Taking inventory of where you've been is the best way to monitor your progress. Knowing what worked best for you (and what didn't) in the past enables you to make clear, empowering choices going forward.

BOMBSHELL BONUS
Soothe Yourself with Scent

Here's a rundown of our favorite soothing essential oils:

- ✱ **Lavender:** This is the ultimate relaxation scent. Lavender reduces inflammation, relieves aches and pains, and promotes deep sleep.
- ✱ **Neroli:** Orange-scented neroli is wonderful for reducing anxiety and relieving headaches.
- ✱ **Vanilla:** This scent is soothing and warming but also has a sexy side: It's known to increase libido!
- ✱ **Ylang-ylang:** When your nerves feel a little fried, use ylang-ylang to set things right and lift your mood.
- ✱ **Lemongrass:** For potent stress relief, add a few drops of lemongrass.

Be Fabulous

Your day of inner reflection ends with a lovely treat . . .

Your BE FABULOUS Challenge:
Get a Little Bubble Therapy

Ahhh . . . nothing beats a delicious soak in a luxurious bath! It's just what a magnificent mermaid like you deserves. So turn off the phone, set the DVR to record your favorite show, and give yourself this gift to soothe your mind and spirit. As a bonus, you'll emerge with silky, sweet-smelling skin.

Here's the recipe for our favorite Tone It Up soak. You'll need:

One of the places I find the most peace is in the shower. There's just something magical about being in water.—Katrina

- 1 cup Epsom salt
- 3 teaspoons moisturizing oil of your choice. Almond, coconut, and jojoba are all excellent options.
- 10 drops essential oil of your choice

Add all the ingredients to a warm bath. The Epsom salt will ease sore muscles, draw out toxins, and promote relaxation. The essential oils can work wonders on your stress, and the oil will leave you with silky-soft skin. So just climb in and let the cares of the day melt away.

Allow your mind to drift. Nothing to do, nowhere to be. Just breathe and relax. Your inner wisdom is right there, waiting for you to quiet down your busy brain and let it emerge. So don't be surprised if you have some big realizations or ideas while you're submerged!

I'm a vanilla girl all the way. It's just so warm and delicious . . . it smells like something yummy baking!—Katrina

Sometimes in the morning, I'll dab eucalyptus oil on my wrists and use some in a spritzer when I'm in the shower, to make my own little spa steam room. I love how it helps me start the day feeling clearheaded and energized.—Karena

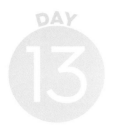

DAY

13

Saturday

Your Word for Today: Light
Your Mantra: I am free, clear, and light.

These 28 days are not just about shedding pounds. They're also for shedding all the junk and clutter that mentally gets in your way and weighs you down. Today you're going to ditch some baggage so you feel free, clear, and wide open to take on anything and everything!

Be Fit

Here is your BE FIT plan for today:

✳ Morning Booty Call

✳ Daily Fitness Challenge:
   HIIT: Shred and Shine (page 221)

✳ Fab Food of the Day:
   Carrots

✳ Body-Loving Recipe of the Day:
   Carrot-Pineapple Slaw

🕐 Your Morning Booty Call

Your goal for this morning: lightness and ease. As you do your Morning Booty Call activity, pay attention to how you step, lift, run, bend, and stretch and make the effort to move with fluidity and grace. Breathe deeply and let your body flow.

Yoga is an excellent way to release tension and tightness that can weigh you down, mentally and physically. Clear your mind, body, and soul for this beautiful day ahead with the Yin Yoga Booty Call routine on page 257.

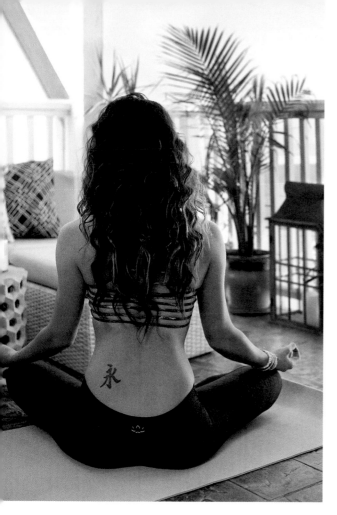

tional benefits. If you want to eat them cooked, lightly steam them.

🍽 Body-Loving Recipe of the Day
Carrot-Pineapple Slaw

This sweet, crunchy slaw is easy to make and jam-packed with flavor and nutrients.

Serves 2

- 1½ cups shredded or shoestring carrots
- ¼ fresh pineapple, diced
- 2 sprigs mint, chopped
- ½ fresh lime, juiced
- 1 teaspoon honey or agave nectar
- ¼ teaspoon sea salt
- ½ teaspoon extra-virgin olive oil
- ¼ cup chopped pistachios

In a medium bowl, mix together the carrots, pineapple, and mint. Add the lime juice, honey or agave, salt, and oil and combine the ingredients thoroughly. Once mixed, top with the pistachios. Chill for 20 minutes before serving.

Be Fierce

Ahhh . . . the key to a clear, focused mind: organization! Our homes are our sanctuary and should be treated that way. A cluttered house equals a cluttered mind. It's time to clear your space of what's weighing you down. Today you're going to rid yourself of the items

🍎 Fab Food of the Day
Carrots

Carrots are rich in antioxidants, vitamins, and minerals, including beta-carotene; potassium; vitamins K, A, and E; magnesium; and zinc. These crunchy powerhouses are known for protecting eyesight, improving liver function, and boosting immunity. Plus, they contain natural sugars that keep you alert and focused. Eating carrots raw provides the most nutri-

I can't work until my surroundings are in place and my house is clean. I call it my 10-minute cleanup in the mornings or at the end of my workday—I'll take 10 to 15 minutes and put stuff away. I figure if I do 10 minutes a day, then when the weekend rolls around, I'm not spending my whole Saturday doing it.—Karena

I'm still working on being organized. I used to have a lot of to-do lists, and I'm starting to do that more. I'm also planning more dinner parties because, honestly, it gets me to clean up the house!—Katrina

you don't need to hold on to anymore so you have plenty of mental (and physical) space to welcome in new possibilities.

Your BE FIERCE Challenge:
Declutter Your Life to Declutter Your Mind

This challenge could take some time, so don't feel you need to do every nook and cranny in your house in one day. It's best to start small and tackle one space at a time. For instance, you could focus just on your kitchen or bathroom and clear a few cabinets, or choose one room to do per day. With each item you come across, ask yourself:

- Do I use this?
- Do I need it?
- Do I genuinely like it?

Unless the answer to all three is yes, out it goes! The bottom line here is that you want to clear away anything that is old, broken, or outdated or that doesn't make you smile or make your life easier. Go through your closet and take out any workout clothes you don't wear anymore—especially if they don't make you feel good when you put them on. There are too many fabulous, stylish options out there to clog up your closet with old, ratty ones! Donate as much as is reusable to your local Goodwill or donation center.

Go through your kitchen and take out every old bottle, spice, and box from the back of the cabinet. If it's expired, toss it. If it's a boxed or canned good you know you'll never use, donate it to a food bank or shelter.

Just keep going through all the corners of your home, one by one. You'll know when

BOMBSHELL BONUS
Get It Together with Your To-Dos

Grab your journal, calendar, or smartphone and start writing out your daily to-dos. These can be anything from things to get done at work, errands to run, calls to make, and dates with friends. This list will now be how you organize your day. Writing things down will help you stay present and focus on your current task, which makes you more productive and calm. When you know what you need to get done and when, your mind is freed up for all the creative brainstorming and big dreaming you're doing!

you're done because you'll feel 10 pounds lighter and *free*!

Be Fabulous

While we're on the topic of shedding, today you're going to exfoliate to reveal your radiant complexion. Exfoliating rejuvenates by sloughing away the dead surface layer that can dull and dry your skin. It also increases circulation, which helps decrease the appearance of cellulite. By the way, the coffee in the super-smoothing scrub you're about to read about does this as well! Caffeine has an anti-inflammatory effect, which makes your skin look tight and smooth.

Your BE FABULOUS Challenge:
Exfoliate for Extra Glow

Here's what you'll need:

- 1½ cups coarsely ground coffee (no decaf!)
- ½ cup sugar or sea salt
- 3 tablespoons melted coconut oil or olive oil

Mix the coffee and sugar or salt together well. Add in the oil and stir until it looks like a thick paste. Toward the end of a warm shower, rub the mixture over your legs, booty, midsection, and arms using firm, circular motions. If you like, you can let the mixture sit for a few minutes before rinsing with warm water for a little extra silkifying (make sure to use a drain mesh to prevent the grounds from clogging your pipes).

For quick exfoliation on days when you don't have time to mix up a batch of DIY

I like to double my batch of coffee scrub and put it into mason jars to give to friends. Tie a ribbon around the jar and you have a pretty gift they'll love!—Katrina

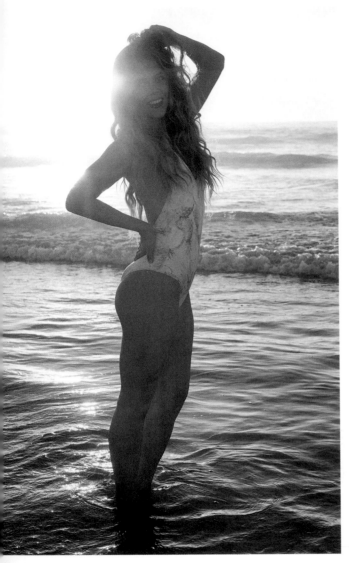

scrub, try dry brushing. Dry brushing is a simple, easy, and inexpensive way to clear pores, improve skin texture (hellooo silky stems and sleek arms!), and reduce the appearance of cellulite. The best thing about dry brushing is that it stimulates the lymphatic system, helping your body detox and get rid of excess fluid. Plus, it's fantastically invigorating and refreshing!

All you need is a high-quality natural bristle brush or loofah. The best time to dry brush is in the morning, before you shower. After your morning workout is ideal! Start low, at your feet, and work your way up using short, firm (but not painful) upward strokes. Move your way up your body, paying close attention to your underarms and neck, where lymph nodes are located. On those areas as well as your tummy, use circular, clockwise strokes. Spend anywhere from 5 to 20 minutes on this daily and you'll see astonishing results!

Sunday

Your Word for Today: Calm
Your Mantra: I am at peace.

Yesss . . . it's Sweet Surrender Sunday! Today you're going to give up the go-go-go and just be-be-be. So hop off the merry-go-round and take this delicious day to unplug, let go of your worries, and find some inner peace.

Be Fit

Here is your BE FIT plan for today:

* Morning Booty Call
* Daily Fitness Challenge:
  Active rest day
* Fab Food of the Day:
  Walnuts
* Body-Loving Recipe of the Day:
  Four-Ingredient Cookies

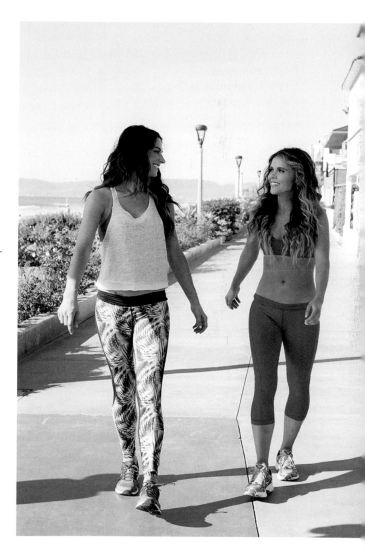

Bonus Recipe

Tipsy Apples and Walnuts

We love an occasional glass of wine, and while we have a fondness for whites, reds are delicious antioxidant powerhouses! Moderate consumption of red wine has been shown to have many benefits, including staving off depression, preventing UV skin damage, and even combating the effects of aging.

You're going to swoon over this deliciously unique mix of some of our favorite flavors. This recipe combines the benefits of red wine with healthy, fresh fruit and omega-3-rich walnuts.

Serves 2

- 1 Gala or Fuji apple
- ¼ fresh lemon, juiced
- ½ cup chopped raw walnuts
- ½ teaspoon ground cinnamon
- ¼ cup raisins
- ½ cup your favorite red wine

Wash the apple and finely dice it into small, bite-size pieces. Immediately after chopping, place the apple pieces in a large bowl and coat them with lemon juice to prevent browning. Add all the other ingredients, stir well, and allow to marinate at room temperature for 15 to 30 minutes prior to serving.

Your Morning Booty Call

Today is a rest day, so take your Morning Booty Call down a notch today from whatever you're accustomed to. Just as you did on Day 5, try something a little slower or gentler, like a walk, stretching, or Yin Yoga (page 257), to give your body and spirit some time to recover.

Don't forget your morning ritual and list of daily nonnegotiables! No matter what—whether you're going all out or taking it easy—these are now an essential part of how you begin your day.

Fab Food of the Day
Walnuts

Food can have a major impact on your mood and your mind-set. Take walnuts, for example. One of the highest natural sources of the all-important, anti-inflammatory omega-3s, walnuts have been shown to help the body respond better to stress. They're also a stealth little source of protein and they help oxidize fats, which encourages weight loss and keeps your peaceful heart happy.

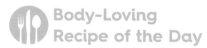

Body-Loving Recipe of the Day

Four-Ingredient Cookies

The best kind of cookie is one you can indulge in anytime with no regrets. And this one's it! It's so simple to make, and with omega-3 fatty acids, protein, fiber, and potassium, this cookie is quite the nutritional knockout!

Serves 2

- 2 medium ripe bananas, peeled
- 1 scoop or packet vanilla Perfect Fit protein powder
- 1 cup rolled oats
- ½ cup crushed walnuts

Preheat the oven to 350°F.

In a medium bowl, thoroughly mash the bananas with a fork. Add the protein powder and keep mixing. If the mixture is too thick to mash well, you may need to add a few drops of almond milk or water to get the dough to the right consistency. Fold in the oats and walnuts.

Coat a cookie sheet with nonstick cooking spray. Using a tablespoon, drop the dough onto the cookie sheet, lightly pressing down on each to flatten (this helps them bake better!). Bake for 15 to 20 minutes, or until golden brown.

Be Fierce

You're probably wondering, "How can I chill out and be fierce at the same time?!" That's easy for a bold, bodacious babe like yourself: by actively and unflinchingly declaring a rest day for yourself! Let your significant other know that you're taking today to restore. Make your kids giggle and tell them mama is taking a pj day. Tell your friends you're chilling at home today. Chances are some or all of them will be so thrilled by the idea, they'll want to do the same!

Your BE FIERCE Challenge: *Do Nothing*

Yes, that's right: We want you to fiercely *do nothing* that is anything other than relaxing and restorative. Sleep in. Watch a movie. Read

My favorite chill-out activity is lying on the beach. I love the hit of warm sunshine and vitamin D, listening the waves, feeling the warm sand between my toes . . . oh, and salty kisses from my husband! In the winter, my best weekend days are staying home with Brian, making soup, and watching a full season of a show we missed with our animals cuddled up next to me.—Katrina

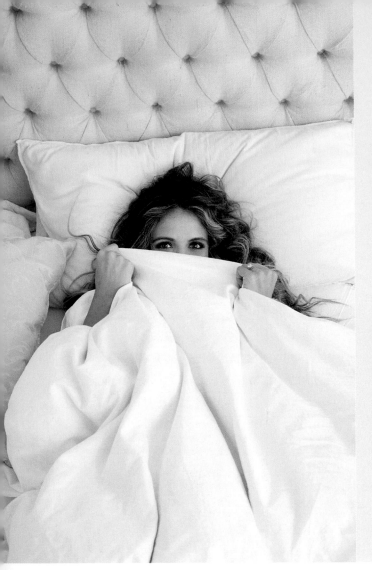

What's your favorite way to relax?

✳ Sitting by the fire, cuddling on the couch, and watching movies with my family.—Kelli R.

✳ Soaking up the sun on my back deck with a glass of wine and my dog. Sometimes I bring my computer and use StumbleUpon to discover new things. I love learning and discovering new stuff!—Kate R.

✳ Going out for coffee with my bestie, going with my boyfriend and dogs to the lake, or just watching television.—Tiffany M.

✳ Anything outdoors that connects me with nature: a hike, a walk, sitting on the beach, playing Frisbee with the kids, even yard work!—Jillian M.

✳ Take a bath! I love picking out a special bath bomb or bath bubbles; I keep a variety in my shower so I can choose a special one each time. It's like a little variety shop of goodies! —Candice M.

✳ Go to a restorative yoga class.—Debbie M.

a book. Go for a leisurely walk or linger at brunch with friends. Shelve your worries just for today. Forget the pressing demands or the problems you need to solve. We promise, with a restored sense of calm from today, you'll be far better equipped to solve them with ease tomorrow.

Be Fabulous

Cell phones ringing. Texts dinging. E-mails pinging. We've gotten so used to being wired in 24/7 that these sounds are as constant and normal to us as our breathing—and that's not necessarily a good thing. All the sounds and stimuli of the modern world are a big disrup-

118 • Tone It Up

tion to our inner peace and quiet. Don't get us wrong—we love our smartphones as much as any of you, trust us! But sometimes we all just need a break to disconnect from the world and reconnect with our calm within.

Your BE FABULOUS Challenge:
Take a Nighttime Tech Detox

From the time you sit down to dinner until you go to bed tonight, power down your cell phone. Close the computer. Turn off the television. Take this evening to calm not just your body and brain but your spirit as well. Unplug from the constant stimulation and just enjoy some peace and quiet tonight. Read a book. Sit and have a conversation with someone you love. Take a bath or indulge in any of your favorite fabulous beauty treats from the last 2 weeks.

On weekends, if the weather is warm, I love to just sit on my front porch and read a magazine. In the winter, sleeping in and watching a movie in bed is just the best.—Karena

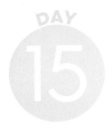

DAY
15

Monday

Your Word for Today: Present
Your Mantra: Today I am awake and aware, moment by moment.

You have somewhere around 1,000 minutes to spend today during your waking hours. How many of those will you really be *awake* for? By "awake," we mean aware and fully present. Today is all about paying attention and getting the most out of each and every precious moment.

Be Fit

Here is your BE FIT plan for today:

* Take and record your measurements.
* Morning Booty Call
* Daily Fitness Challenge:
  Full-Body Toning: Bombshell Bonanza
  (page 204)
* Fab Food of the Day: Miso
* Body-Loving Recipe of the Day:
  Sautéed Tempeh with Sesame-Ginger
  Dressing

Take and Record Your Measurements

Look at you, getting tighter and slimmer by the day! Repeat your measure-and-record process today. Go ahead . . . we know you want to share those incredible results with the Tone It Up community, and they (and we) really want to hear about them! Post a photo or news of your accomplishments to #FitFierceFab.

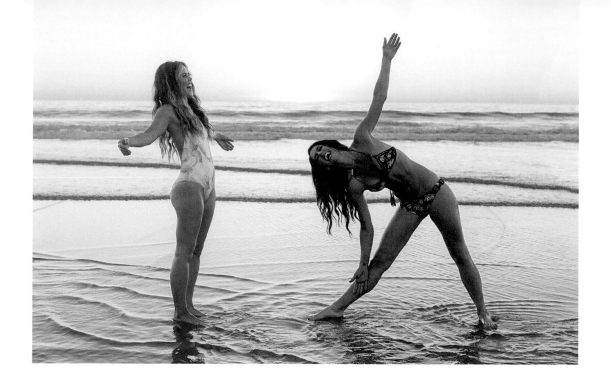

Your Morning Booty Call

Wake up, sleeping beauty! And we don't just mean by opening your eyes and rolling out of bed. Today is a day for all kinds of awakening, which starts with being fully engaged and present with everyone and everything around you. We'll get to your full-on BE FIERCE challenge of being present in a minute, but for now, just tune in and pay attention—*really* pay attention—to the small details of your morning routine. Even if it's something you've done a million times before, like brushing your teeth or walking the dog. Don't just go through the motions; really notice what you see, hear, smell, taste, and feel. Taste the minty freshness of the toothpaste, feel your doggie's soft fur, breathe in the sweet morning air, listen to the sounds of the world waking up all around you. You'll likely be surprised by how many spectacular sensations you've been missing out on.

I've learned that the little pockets of full presence are so important. These moments in which we're fully awake and taking life in are what it's all about.—Karena

Fab Food of the Day
Miso

Made from fermented soybeans, miso contains valuable living enzymes that keep your digestive system running at maximum efficiency. These enzymes help restore the good bacteria in your gut—the ones that keep you slim and bloat-free. It comes in a red or white paste you can find at your local health food store or Whole Foods. Just a little dab of either variety adds a delicious salty flavor to dishes.

Body-Loving Recipe of the Day

Sautéed Tempeh with Sesame-Ginger Dressing

With a sweet, Asian-inspired dressing, this is tempeh's time to shine! Pair this dish with your favorite steamed veggies like broccoli, bok choy, and carrots.

Serves 2

Sautéed Tempeh

- ½ teaspoon sesame oil
- 4 ounces tempeh
- 2 cups greens of your choice (we suggest broccoli or bok choy)
- ¼ cup grated or chopped carrot

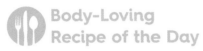

Tantalizing Tip

Look for organic, unpasteurized miso paste for the most potent benefits.

Dressing

- 2 tablespoons carrot juice or orange juice
- 1½ tablespoons white miso
- 1½ tablespoons sesame oil
- 1 tablespoon toasted sesame seeds
- 1½ tablespoons rice vinegar
- 1 piece fresh ginger (1½ inches), grated
- 1 clove garlic, minced

Heat a pan on medium-high and add the oil. Add the tempeh and greens; sauté for 4 to 5 minutes. Add the carrot and toss for another 2 minutes. Remove from the heat.

In a bowl, whisk together the juice, miso, oil, seeds, vinegar, ginger, and garlic. Drizzle the dressing over the tempeh and vegetable mixture and enjoy!

Be Fierce

You've already started your day on the right track. Now we're going to keep that going and dedicate today to being fully, blissfully awake and present.

Your BE FIERCE Challenge:
Live in the Moment

Today we want you to make a conscious effort to be and stay aware in every moment. Appreciate what is going on right now in front of you and around you. Take the time to enjoy the sweet moments of laughing with a friend, tasting a delicious dish, seeing a stunning sunset. When you have a conversation with someone, pay extra attention and really listen to what they are saying. Look them in the eye (yes . . . you remember this challenge). Take in what's going on right now—not what happened at that meeting this morning or what you'll cook for dinner this evening.

If you find yourself getting off track and zoning out, thinking about what happened yesterday or what will happen tomorrow, use your senses to snap you out of it. They're your instantaneous ticket back to the right here and now. What do you see, hear, smell, feel, taste? It's impossible to zone out and fully tune in to your senses at the same time, and that'll wake you right up.

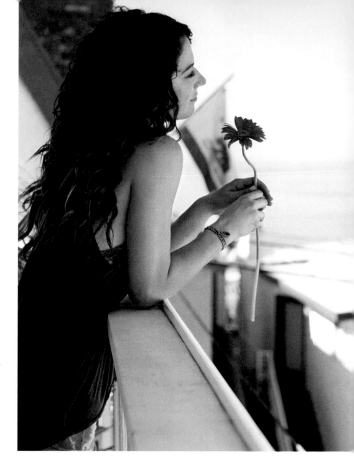

BOMBSHELL BONUS
Shake It Up to Wake It Up!

Want a fast and easy way to shut off the autopilot mode? Change up your usual routine. The same old, same old lets us mentally snooze, but the unfamiliar keeps you on your toes. If you walk or drive the same route to work every day, your brain automatically steers you. So go a different way today! If you always eat the same thing for breakfast, it's easy to prepare it without really noticing you're doing it. So whip up something out of the ordinary this morning. Go to the 8:30 barre class at a different studio instead of the 9:15 at your usual joint. Give your regular a rest and see what happens.

Be Fabulous

Let's talk about your sexy, sassy mane. Do you wear your hair the same way nearly every day? Join the club. Your tried-and-true style probably looks great on you. But just for today, we challenge you to give a different 'do a whirl. Trust us, you'll capture your full attention every time you look in the mirror today!

Your BE FABULOUS Challenge:
Do a New 'Do

Sport a sleek ponytail. Flash some flirty curls. Wow 'em with a sophisticated updo. Today's the day to mix things up and try on a new look. Who knows? You might discover a new fave to work into your usual rotation.

Speaking of faves, here are four styles we love to play with . . .

Beachy Waves

Okay, beach babe! This is the secret to getting those beautiful, fun-in-the-sun, sexy curls that everyone from surfers to sailors will swoon over.

For straight hair:

- Wash and blow-dry upside down, then smooth with a round brush.

- Divide hair into top and bottom, then again into 2-inch sections.

- Spritz each section with hair spray. Then,

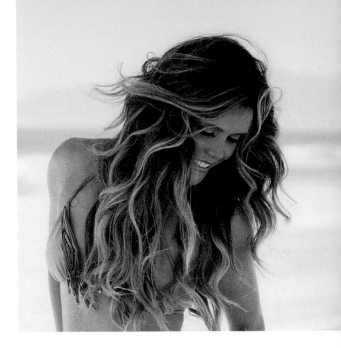

using a curling iron, curl each section away from your face (direction is important!). Be sure to keep the ends off the iron; you want the ends to be straight.

- Spritz your curl with hair spray to hold it, then, when all the curls are done, add your favorite sea salt spray. This will give it amazing texture.

- Flip your head upside down one more time and gently blow-dry the roots, scrunching your hair. This will loosen the curl and give it that natural, bouncy, "I just came from the beach" look!

For naturally curly or wavy hair:

- Flip wet hair upside down and scrunch with a cotton T-shirt.

- Add a small palmful of mousse.

- Spritz with sea salt spray and let air-dry. You still want your ends to be a little straight, so keep running your hands through the ends.

- When it's almost totally dry, flip your hair upside down once more and dry the roots and curls gently with a blow-dryer.

- Touch up the curls around your face following the instructions above.

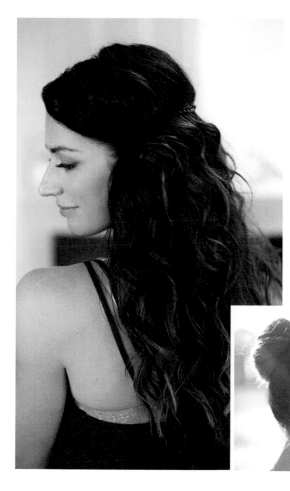

Pretty in Pins

If you're used to wearing your hair down all the time, this is the perfect look to pull it back and show that gorgeous face. Here's how to do it:

- Style your hair as you normally do (or with your beach waves!).

- Part your hair down the middle.

- Take a section from the front of one side of your hairline and twist, pulling it toward the back of your head; secure with two bobby pins.

- Repeat on the other side.

- Bonus: Create two small braids in the front hairline to pull back.

Bun o' Fun

This is a fabulous, quick updo that's great when you're in a hurry. We also love to rock this on hot days.

- Pull all your hair upward on the top of your head into a high ponytail and secure with an elastic band.

  - Use a comb to tease the hair and create messy volume and fluff!

  - Twist the hair around the elastic in a circular motion.

  - Secure the bun with a couple hairpins.

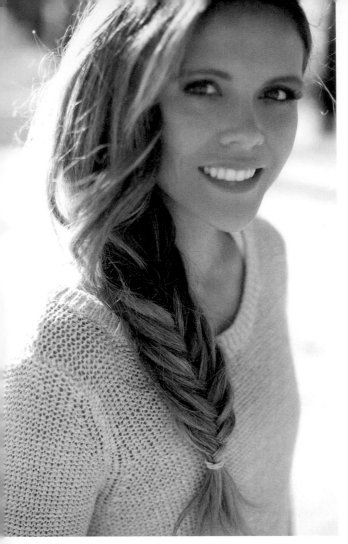

Boho Braids

This style works best with long, textured hair. If your hair is straight, add some texture by adding a few waves (see Beachy Waves on page 124), then follow these steps:

- Gather the hair on one side in a low ponytail.

- Separate the pony into two sections.

- Holding one section of the pony, use your other hand to take a narrow piece of hair from the outside of the other section and cross it over to the inside of the section in your other hand.

- Repeat this on the other side, crossing hair from one section into the other until you run out of hair.

- Secure the end with an elastic band.

- For a looser, more casual look, gently pull the braid apart with your fingers.

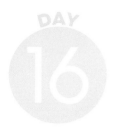

DAY 16

Tuesday

Your Word for Today: Generous
Your Mantra: I give openly and freely from my heart.

Everything you've been doing up until now has been to make you feel empowered, centered, and shining with positive energy. Today you're going to share that beautiful positivity with the world. The amazing thing is that when we give, we end up getting so much more in return.

Be Fit

Here is your BE FIT plan for today:

* Morning Booty Call

* Daily Fitness Challenge:
  Cardio: Fly Me to the Moon (page 244)

* Fab Food of the Day:
  Berries

* Body-Loving Recipe of the Day:
  Berry Blast Detox Smoothie

Your Morning Booty Call

Who in your life could use a little motivation or company as they start their day? Today invite someone to join you for your Morning Booty Call and share the hit of energy you get from it. Bring along your honey on your morning walk, roll out an extra yoga mat for your kids, or call a friend and ask her to come along for whatever workout you're doing. Maybe even share some of the challenges you've done over the past 2 weeks to inspire them to be their own version of Fit, Fierce, and Fabulous!

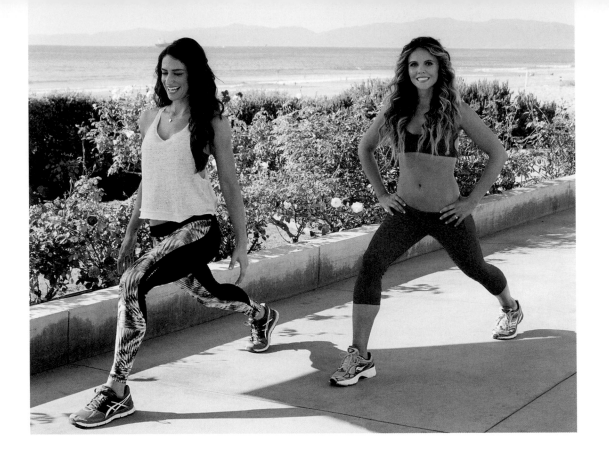

Fab Food of the Day
Berries

Berries symbolize abundance, which is exactly the state of mind you are cultivating today. You have so much to give! These sweet and sassy flavor bombs top the list of high- antioxidant foods (especially blueberries) as well as high-fiber digestive helpers. And strawberries in particular have been shown to do your big, giving heart a lot of good.

Tantalizing Tip

Even if they're in season this time of year, stock up on a few bags of frozen organic berries so you have them on hand to throw into smoothies—or just pop them into your mouth for a quick snack.

Add a scoop of Perfect Fit protein powder to your smoothie if you're enjoying this postworkout.

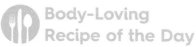

Body-Loving Recipe of the Day
Berry Blast Detox Smoothie

This baby is packed with vitamins, antioxidants, enzymes, and a whole lot of delicious berry goodness.

Serves 2

- 16 ounces coconut water
- 1 frozen peeled banana, sliced
- 2 cups kale, stems removed (*note:* if you have a high-speed blender, you may leave the stems in)
- 1 cup blueberries, fresh or frozen
- 1 cup strawberries, fresh or frozen

Combine all ingredients in a blender and process until smooth.

Be Fierce

Generosity makes us bigger, and anything that expands us makes us stronger. Being generous is often a very bold move. It requires us to offer something of ourselves, and that taps your confidence and makes you feel more connected and present. Bringing someone an unexpected gift, giving a heartfelt compliment to an acquaintance, giving up your seat on the bus to a stranger . . . these are all acts of self-lessness that require you to bravely and directly reach out to another person.

Have you ever had someone do something kind for no reason? Maybe a friend gave you a card to say they care or someone brought you fresh-baked muffins (Tone It Up approved, of course!). However big or small, these things don't go unnoticed. A simple gift from the heart can instantly change someone else's perspective or lift their mood.

Today you're going to discover just how empowering and enriching acts of generosity and kindness can be—for them and for you.

Your BE FIERCE Challenge: *Give It Up*

In yoga the highest form of spirituality is being of service to others. Today reach for the stars and find as many ways to help others as you can. Be selfless—all day. You don't have to make big, sweeping gestures; every act of kindness counts!

Here are just a few examples to get your generosity muscle in gear:

- Make a special breakfast for your roomies.
- Vacuum or pick up the groceries . . . even if it isn't your turn.

- Open doors for people.
- Take out your neighbor's trash.
- Bring a meal to a homeless person you pass.
- Buy a cup of coffee for someone in line behind you.
- Visit an elderly person you know who could use some company.
- Drive a friend to the airport.
- Overtip a service person.
- Go with your special guy or friend to that zombie flick he's been wanting to see.
- Send someone you love a funny or encouraging card.

Open your heart and your eyes and you'll find opportunities everywhere to be your most gorgeous, giving, generous self.

Be Fabulous

By now you've probably figured out that generosity is all about connecting deeply with others, which increases your fabulosity. So how about we go even bigger? Today we challenge you to open your heart even wider and share something special with your #FitFierceFab sisters!

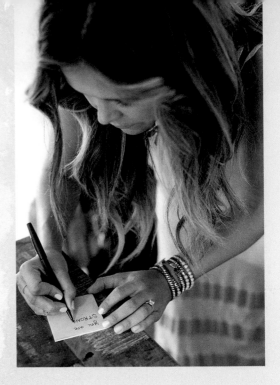

BOMBSHELL BONUS
Surprise Someone

Leave an inspiring note for a stranger in a public place today. You can write it in chalk on the sidewalk, on a sticky note attached to a park bench, or tape up a piece of paper on the back of a restroom door. We like to go with something simple and sweet like "You're amazing!" or "Have a beautiful day!" No, you won't get to see their reaction, but you'll spend today secretly knowing you made someone else smile.

Your BE FABULOUS Challenge:
Share Your Favorite Tone It Up Recipes

What have you been cooking up over there in your kitchen, you culinary goddess? Your Fit, Fierce, and Fabulous sisters want to know!

Today we're asking you to be generous with your creativity and share any new recipes you've come up with. If you loved making and eating it, imagine how many other gals will too! Check in with the Fit, Fierce, and Fabulous group in the Tone It Up community at ToneItUp.com with photos of your recipes and on Instagram, Twitter, and Facebook with hashtag #FitFierceFab and tag @ToneItUp.

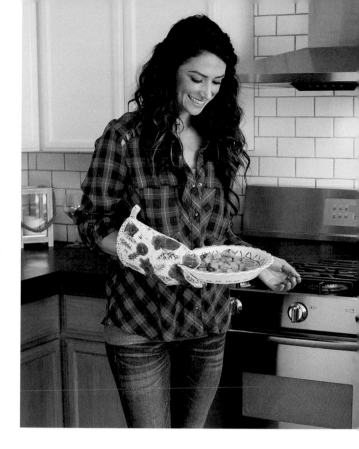

For Valentine's Day this year, I sent all my girlfriends a little Valentine's box. They loved it. It really made their day!—Katrina

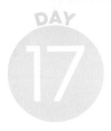

DAY

17

Wednesday

Your Word for Today: Accepting
Your Mantra: I flow easily with everything that comes my way.

Life is happening . . . constantly. Each one of us will experience the ebbs and flows like a wave. Today we'll focus on just staying on the wave and learning to enjoy the ride, no matter what comes our way.

Be Fit

Here is your BE FIT plan for today:

✴ Morning Booty Call

✴ Daily Fitness Challenge: HIIT: Rev Up and Rock Out (page 228)

✴ Fab Food of the Day: Chia seeds

✴ Body-Loving Recipe of the Day: Ginger-Peach Pudding Parfait

Your Morning Booty Call

As you are movin' and groovin' your body this morning, notice if you have moments of wishing that you felt, looked, or moved differently than you do. And then LET IT GO! You're perfect, beautiful, and strong exactly as you are.

Fab Food of the Day
Chia Seeds

These tiny-but-mighty seeds are high in omega-3s as well as vitamins, antioxidants, minerals, and fiber. When you put them in liquid, they create a hydrating gel that is great as a thickener in smoothies or puddings. This gel also sweeps your intestines like a mini internal cleaning crew. Oh, and did we mention that even a small amount is *super* filling?

Body-Loving Recipe of the Day
Ginger-Peach Pudding Parfait

Who says peaches and cream have to be innocent? For a sassy take on this classic combo, whip up this treat for breakfast or dessert or enjoy it as an afternoon pick-me-up.

Serves 2

- 1 cup unsweetened almond milk
- 1 scoop vanilla Perfect Fit protein powder
- 3 tablespoons chia seeds
- 1 teaspoon grated fresh ginger
- 1 cup diced peaches (preferably fresh, if they're in season; otherwise use organic canned peaches without sugar added, drained, or organic frozen peaches)
- ½ cup your favorite granola (stick with all-natural, low-sugar varieties)
- ¼ cup unsweetened shredded coconut

In a blender or shaker bottle, combine the almond milk with the protein powder until smooth. Mix in the chia seeds and ginger and place in the refrigerator overnight.

In the morning, layer the chia pudding with peaches, granola, and coconut.

Be Fierce

One of the most difficult things in life is to accept that sh-t is gonna happen. Nobody ever wants to experience sadness, frustration, pain, or loss, but these are all part of life, and we can't just resist them. The answer is not to throw your hands in the air kicking and screaming. We've all tried that, and other than the momentary release of steam, where does it really get you?

To get to acceptance, we need to change our perspective. You may not be able to control what happens to and around you (we so get it . . . we wish we could too!), but you *can* control how your mind reacts to it. It's not

Tantalizing Tip

Chia seeds are notorious for sticking between teeth, so you may want to do a quick check of your pearly whites after enjoying this treat to be sure your dazzling smile is seed-free!

I always use the saying "It is what it is" and then move
forward into solution.—Karena

always easy—it takes practice—but with your foundation of fierceness, you can do it. Instead of feeling defeated, find a solution. Instead of holding on to something that has hurt you emotionally, free yourself and learn to let go. We can't change what has already happened, but we can control how we respond to the situation and what happens next.

Your BE FIERCE Challenge:
Be Where You Are

No matter what challenges you today, aim to resist reacting with frustration or anger.

When the upset rises up, find something to tell yourself to help you accept what's happening. The trick is to find the mantra of acceptance that works for you. For instance, maybe one of these:

- I flow easily with everything that comes my way.
- This too shall pass.
- Being angry/frustrated/upset doesn't help this situation; only a change in how I see it will release me.
- I will figure this out; I always do.

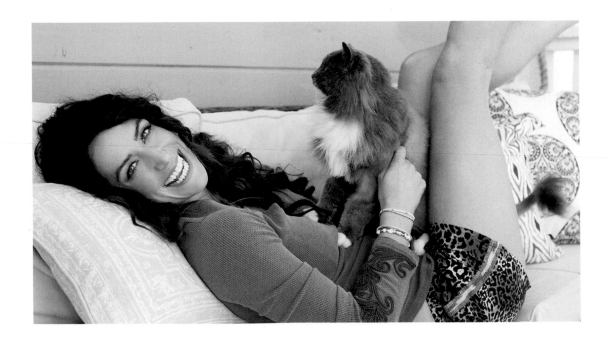

BOMBSHELL BONUS
Accept Your Past

Everything that has happened to you in life up until now has made you into the fierce tigress you are today. From here on out, vow to appreciate every experience and lesson that comes your way—yes, even the challenging ones—because they only make you more A-MAAA-ZZZING!

- I will find peace with this situation. Maybe not today, but soon.
- Everything that happens is here to teach me something valuable that will make me stronger, wiser, deeper.
- This is challenging, but I've worked my way through bigger challenges than this.
- No drama. It's not worth the aggravation!

Start by learning to let go of the little things and it will carry over into more difficult times. We promise if you spend less time worrying and more time simply being and accepting where you are, you will learn to ride that wave with grace and ease.

Be Fabulous

Essential to being fabulous is actually *accepting* that you're fabulous! We can tell you on every single page how strong and beautiful you are, but if you don't let that in and accept it as truth, they're just words.

Today we want you to do something that's hard for most of us, but we know you're up for the challenge.

Your BE FABULOUS Challenge:
Make Peace with All Your Parts

Your mission for today is to accept your gorgeous body, with all its curves, features, strengths, and vulnerabilities. That's right—all of it. There may be things you wish were longer, leaner, higher, smoother, or whatever else, but just for today, you're going to let yourself be and declare, "I am fabulous just the way I am!"

Focusing on all the positive things I have in my life helps me deal with the tough stuff—the good balances out the bad. I look at all the people and experiences I am grateful for and it brings things into perspective.—Katrina

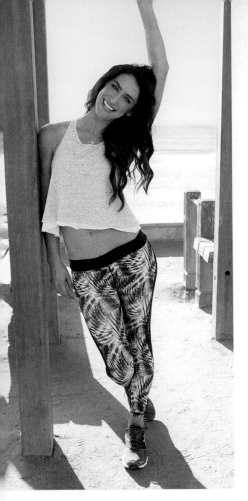

A Little Love from Karena

I have a confession: I have cellulite. Yup. Dimples on the derriere, lumps and bumps on the back of my thighs. A lot of women have this, whether they're in killer shape or not. Ever since I met Kat, who has the best booty EVER, I've worked hard to get it to look like hers. But no matter how many deadlifts or lunges I do, it still doesn't. Does it look better? Absolutely. Is it perfect? No way (who's defining "perfect," anyway?).

But I've learned to work with what I have. I dry brush and use self-tanner to make my rear view look the best it possibly can, and then I just go with what I've got. Up until 7 years ago, I would never wear short shorts because I was afraid of what people would think. Now I rock them because I have the confidence that comes from taking care of myself . . . plus a healthy dose of fierce self-acceptance. Sometimes you've just gotta say, "So what?"

So take it from me: Flaunt it, no matter what. If someone is judging you, that's their problem, not yours! You're healthy, you're in shape, and you're taking fantastic care of yourself, inside and out. You're Fit, Fierce, and Fabulous, and anyone who has a thing to say about a dimple on the back of your thigh clearly just doesn't get it!

Trust us, we're not suggesting this lightly. This is something we work hard to do too . . .

All you're doing in this program is going to get you in *your* best shape, and for that, you deserve a major standing ovation! And, like Karena said, there will also be things you can't change and simply have to accept. Those so-called "flaws" ultimately don't matter, and if you can't change them, why worry about them? You are on your way to creating your most rockin' body—the imperfections are what make you unique and all that much more interesting and BE-YOU-TIFUL! You're an incomparable knockout, babe. Own it.

On that note, we'll leave you with a little xo from Kat:

Today is the youngest you'll ever be and the oldest you've ever been. So right now is the time to wear a frickin' bikini! In 20 years, you'll look back and wish you'd done it, so why wait?!

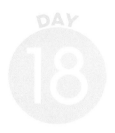
DAY
18

Thursday

Your Word for Today: Forgiving
Your Mantra: Letting go of grudges sets me free.

Just when you thought you cleared the acceptance hurdle with yourself, we're going to challenge you to one more: accepting others with all their flaws and human imperfections. If you can do this—and we know you can—you'll have the unshakable self-assurance that comes from knowing you can rise above anything.

Be Fit

Here is your BE FIT plan for today:

* Morning Booty Call

* Daily Fitness Challenge:
  Full-Body Toning: Bombshell Bonanza
  (page 204)

* Fab Food of the Day: Fennel

* Body-Loving Recipe of the Day:
  Shaved Brussels Sprouts and Fennel Salad

Your Morning Booty Call

Today, either before or during your morning ritual, take a few moments to close your eyes, breathe deeply, and bring your awareness to your chest. Expand as you breathe in lightness to that area and breathe out negativity and rigidity. Imagine your heart warming and softening and hold that image in your mind throughout your day today.

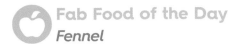

Fab Food of the Day
Fennel

Just like it's good to release old grudges and negative energy, it's good to let go of what we think things "should" taste like and mix things up now and then in the taste-buds department. Fennel is a surefire way to get a little sass into your veggie routine. It has a light, slightly sweet flavor with a hint of anise and is delicious roasted, in salads, or even juiced! Plus, it's rich in fiber, vitamin C, potassium, and phytonutrients that give it antioxidant properties.

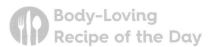

Body-Loving Recipe of the Day

Shaved Brussels Sprouts and Fennel Salad

You can never go wrong with a crisp, fresh salad bursting with interesting flavors, and this one is no exception! It makes a delectable side dish for any occasion or a filling main event when paired with lean protein.

Serves 2

Salad

- 1 cup Brussels sprouts, shaved or thinly sliced
- ¼ cup fennel, shaved or thinly sliced
- 4 dates, sliced

Golden Sun Dressing

- ½ cup fresh lemon juice
- ½ tablespoon minced fresh garlic
- 2 teaspoons honey
- Sea salt, to taste
- 1 tablespoon extra-virgin olive oil

Blanch the Brussels sprouts in hot water for 3 minutes. Remove from the water and let cool for a few minutes, then mix with the fennel and dates.

In a medium bowl, whisk together all the dressing ingredients except the oil. Once well blended, add the oil and whisk for approximately 2 minutes. Drizzle the dressing over the salad and enjoy!

Tantalizing Tip

Add some shredded chicken and a handful of slivered almonds to the Brussels sprouts and fennel salad and voilà! You've got an easy and uniquely satisfying meal.

Be Fierce

Forgiving those who have hurt or offended you is an important step in building your inner strength. It takes real courage to let go. If there is forgiveness to be done, today you'll take the brave step out of your comfort zone and stand face-to-face with your fears. That's what being FIERCE is all about.

Your BE FIERCE Challenge:
Call a Truce

Think of one person in your life against whom you're holding a grudge. Maybe it's a coworker you had a disagreement with, a family member who did something hurtful, or a girlfriend you got into a catfight with. As you think of them (and you want to focus on them, not on the details of what happened; reliving the story will only kick up the anger all over again), call to mind that beautiful sensation from this morning of your soft, open, expansive heart. That was the feeling of compassion that will release you.

The secret to forgiveness is to remember

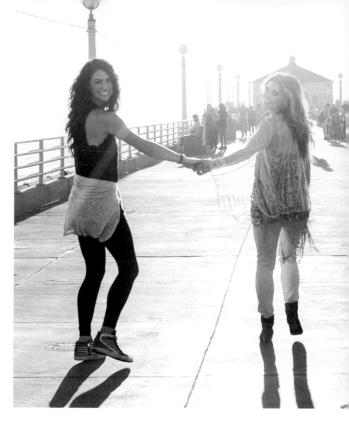

that we're all perfectly imperfect. Everyone is doing the best they can with the resources they have, even if it doesn't match your standards. Fill your heart with love and release the judgment and negativity you're holding on to. Forgive them and move on! It doesn't mean that what they did was okay, or even that you have to let them back into your life. You're

My dad is a therapist by day and a songwriter by night. He has this song called "Love Always Wins" that always stuck with me. I think in everything we do, we need to show up with love. In order to love always, you have to forgive.—Karena

BOMBSHELL BONUS
Love Always Wins

Here's Karena's favorite snippet from her dad Nick Ivanovich's amazing and inspiring song:

So many mysteries in the stars above,
But you can never escape the reach of love
Cause love always wins.
Even after the last whisper of the night has been silenced
Cause love always wins.
Even after the final episode of the ravages of violence
Cause love always wins.

choosing to let go of the negative feelings for yourself, not for them. You are the one who has the power to keep your beautiful heart open no matter what—so use it!

By the way, this forgiveness thing runs both ways. A lot of us have relationships that have gone astray because of something that we've done (or something we haven't done). If there's something you need to apologize for, today's the day to do it. Pick up the phone, write a letter, send an e-mail, and with honor and grace, apologize. No excuses, no defenses.

Just let them know you are sorry for what transpired and, if it's appropriate, that you love them. It's hard, but it will release you.

Be Fabulous

Forgiveness is fierce in that it takes courage. But it's also pretty fabulous, because there's nothing more beautiful than an open heart.

Your BE FABULOUS Challenge: *Let It Slide*

Make today a day of compassion. That means that when the barista at the coffee shop is moving slower than you'd like, give him or her a break; they're probably doing the best they can. If your coworker takes up 15 minutes of your valuable time relaying the details of her dog's stomach virus, just smile and listen; she's probably looking to connect with you. If your sweetie leaves his socks on the floor, simply pick them up and put them in the laundry; no harm, no foul. You likely have habits that drive him crazy too. All day, just let go of all those annoying, irritating, maddening things that usually get you going. Take off the boxing gloves, dial down the impatience, and just allow yourself to soften. Save your fierceness for all the positive challenges we're giving you!

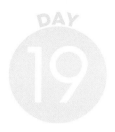

Friday

Joyful
Head up. Shoulders back. Heart open.

Calling all bombshells: It's party time! Today kicks off your weekend, so let's stir up some happy!

Be Fit

Here is your BE FIT plan for today:

* Morning Booty Call
* Daily Fitness Challenge: Cardio: Fly Me to the Moon (page 244)
* Fab Food of the Day: Cacao (aka chocolate!)
* Body-Loving Recipe of the Day: Chocolate-Almond-Banana Smoothie

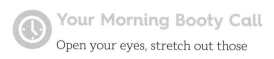

Your Morning Booty Call

Open your eyes, stretch out those sleepy muscles, and before you put one foot on the floor, SMILE. Just the act of raising the corners of your mouth will release some of those happy endorphins to kick off your day with a delicious dose of joy.

What activity do you genuinely love to do? Ride your bike? Go for a run at sunrise? Give a little extra TLC to that fab booty of yours with the Booty Shorts routine on page 251? Whatever it is, today's definitely the day to start off with something that makes you feel good. Now, get out there and get ready to sweat, tone, and have a blast!

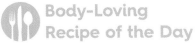 Fab Food of the Day
Cacao (aka Chocolate!)

It's not all in your head that chocolate makes you happy! Studies show that the phytochemicals in cocoa powder can actually improve our mood and make us feel good. This sweet treat also contains sky-high levels of antioxidants that keep your skin radiant. A food that makes us feel good *and* look good? Yes, please!

Add cacao powder or nibs to smoothies or baked goods or whip up some healthy hot chocolate. Or use it in the get-happy recipe below.

Body-Loving Recipe of the Day
Chocolate-Almond-Banana Smoothie

Sometimes the simplest things in life are the sweetest . . .

Serves 2

- 1 frozen peeled banana, sliced
- 2 cups unsweetened vanilla almond milk
- 1 scoop (or 1 packet) Perfect Fit protein powder
- 2 tablespoons cacao nibs

In a blender, place all ingredients and blend until smooth.

Be Fierce

Ohhh, lovelies, have we got some fun fierceness in store for you today!

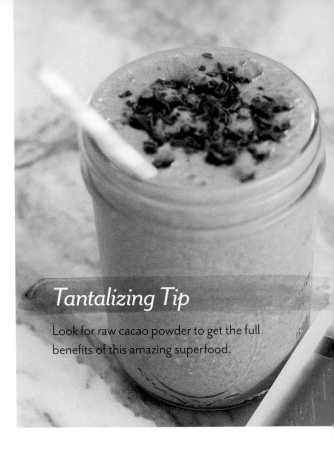

Tantalizing Tip

Look for raw cacao powder to get the full benefits of this amazing superfood.

Your BE FIERCE Challenge:
Sing Your Heart Out

Sounds strange, but this is so liberating! We do it all the time. We've had many long days that end with blasting our favorite song in the car on the way home and singing at the top of our lungs. It's so freeing to sing out loud and proud! Music is a fantastic way to release tension and turn up the joy dial to eleven. You might feel uncomfortable at the beginning, but we promise, you'll finish with a huge laugh or smile. Sing in the shower, in the car, in your living room . . . wherever you can really belt it out!

In case you need a little inspiration to get

I love soothing colors that remind me of the ocean, like teals and dark blues. My entire home reflects my love of the beach.—Karena

you going, take a song from our get-happy playlist to sing along to:

- "7/11" by Beyoncé
- "Come Get It Bae" by Pharrell Williams
- "Chandelier" by Sia
- "Latch" by Disclosure
- "Burn" by Ellie Goulding

For more musical inspiration, go to ToneItUp.com to check out our full playlists—as well as kick-ass ones from Tone It Up members everywhere!

Be Fabulous

We all know joy comes from within—no question there. It's a feeling we get deep in our hearts and souls. But you know what? Joy is also something we can surround ourselves with so it floods into our souls, and that's exactly what you're about to do.

For any of you who read our blog, you know how near and dear to our hearts decorating is! We believe every girl deserves a blissful, beautiful, personal sanctuary. So today we're going to share our secrets for making your magical mermaid cove a space that reflects all that is fabulous and unique about you!

Your BE FABULOUS Challenge: *Make Your Home a Happy Haven*

You don't have to go into full-on renovation mode to make your home into a palace of fabulosity. It's all about making it personal and special to *you*. Most of the time it's the small touches that make the biggest difference.

Here are our favorite tips for creating joy in your home:

- Surround yourself with colors you love. Are you mad for crimson? Passionate about purple? Whatever your signature shade is, use it liberally around your home.

I don't know what it is about soft colors lately, but my eye is drawn to pale shades. Karena adds the color in my life, and I brighten her day with faded blues, whites, and creams.—Katrina

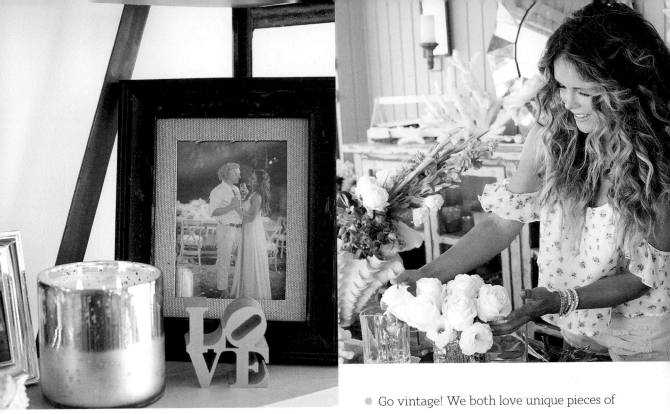

Color has a powerful effect on our mood, as you already learned on Day 8.

- Frame photos of your favorite people and places and display them where you can see them. You'll smile every time you pass by one.

- Fill your home with things that have personal meaning to you.

- Go vintage! We both love unique pieces of vintage furniture and art that have a story. They have such soul. We like to fantasize about who owned them, what kind of joy they brought to other people's homes, and all the things they went through together. It's kind of romantic.

- Buy some fresh flowers to put in your home. They're an inexpensive way to instantly generate joy. A study published in the *Journal of Evolutionary Psychology*

I have my grandmother's paintings up on my walls. These are special to me, because she's the one who introduced me to painting. They're also a daily reminder that what you create in this world can last through generations of family. I hope my granddaughter has some of my artwork in her home someday!—Katrina

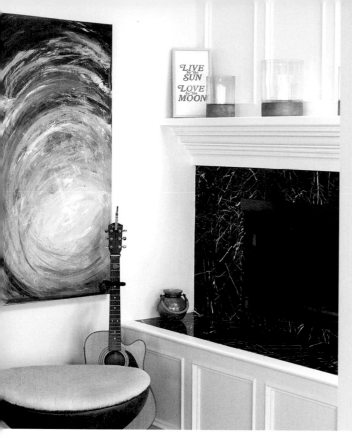

What's in your home that makes it feel like a happy haven?

✻ Pictures. I love all of the experiences I've been through in my life and I love to look back and see those colorful, cheerful memories.—Kate R.

✻ Candles, fresh flowers, and a giant soft blanket.—Stephanie F.

✻ My three pups.—Krystie S.

✻ Shelves filled with books I've read and loved. —Ava G.

✻ My inspiration area, where I keep my inspiration board, yoga mat, and many more special items. I highly recommend everyone have a little inspiration nook they can visit whenever they want to feel happy!—Candice M.

showed that fresh flowers do indeed trigger feelings of happiness.

● Place scented candles around. This one is a must for Karena! The first thing she does every day as part of her morning ritual is light her grapefruit-scented candle in the summer or pumpkin spice in the winter.

● Make memories. This is probably what most makes a house into a joyful home! Gather your friends together for dinner in your home. Celebrate holidays with your family there. Open your home to the people who matter most to you, and they in turn will fill it with love.

I purchased a lot of the decor for my wedding so I could have it in my home after. Brian and I have beautiful reminders of our special day in almost every room: vintage sea glass bottles, dried coral, table runners that my mom made, and centerpieces. The loveseat that we sat on that day is in our bedroom.—Katrina

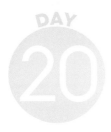
Saturday

Your Word for Today: Frisky
Your Mantra: Ooh la la . . . I'm feelin' FINE!

'fris-kē\\: playful or lively

   Synonyms: bouncy, bubbly, active, animated, zestful, spirited, zippy, peppy, bright-eyed, frolicsome

   See where we're headed with this? Today's your day to release your inner wild child!

Be Fit

Here is your BE FIT plan for today:

* Morning Booty Call

* Daily Fitness Challenge:
  HIIT: Rev Up and Rock Out (page 228)

* Fab Food of the Day:
  Cayenne pepper

* Body-Loving Recipe of the Day:
  Spicy Chickpea Patties

Your Morning Booty Call

   Hey there, you frisky fox. Open your eyes and say helloooo to your sassy Saturday!

Fab Food of the Day
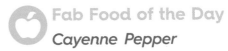
Cayenne Pepper

Kick up those heels, senoritas—things are about to get *spicy!*

   Hot peppers contain a compound called capsaicin, which is known to regulate body temperature, improve circulation, and put the kibosh on an out-of-control appetite. Some studies have even shown that this spicy sensation can help your body burn more calories!

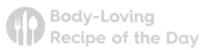

Body-Loving Recipe of the Day

Spicy Chickpea Patties

Unlike the bland veggie burger you've come to know, this bright, flavorful patty will knock your spicy socks off!

Serves 2

- ½ 15-ounce can organic, no-salt-added chickpeas, rinsed, drained, and mashed
- 2 tablespoons grated carrots
- ¼ onion, minced
- 2 tablespoons ground flaxseed
- ½ teaspoon paprika
- ½ teaspoon cumin powder
- ½ teaspoon turmeric powder
- ½ teaspoon cayenne pepper

In a bowl, thoroughly combine all ingredients. If the mixture is too crumbly, add water slowly (1 tablespoon at a time) until it reaches a smooth yet firm consistency.

Form the mixture into 2 burger-size patties. Grill for about 3 minutes on each side or place in a greased skillet (we like using organic cooking spray or a little bit of grape seed oil) and cook until evenly browned.

Serve with a 100% whole wheat bun or on portobello mushrooms with your favorite healthy condiments.

Be Fierce

Laughing and having fun is ultimately what this is all for. Why do all this work if you're not going to enjoy the results? We don't just want you to look and feel your best—we want you to be able to appreciate it! You're light, you're present, you're joyful . . . now use that positive energy to love up the great big world out there. There are so many incredible things waiting for you to see, taste, and try.

We *loooove* a good adventure—especially one that leaves lots of room for spontaneity. Last summer we took a trip to Europe with not much more than our guys, a loose itinerary, and an "oh heck yes let's try it" attitude. We didn't know what we were going to discover each day when we set out, and all the new things and experiences we encountered were so eye-opening. We wandered the

Tantalizing Tip

Be sure to read labels on any extras you jazz up your chickpea patties with, like ketchup, sauces, and so on. If they contain high fructose corn syrup or other scary-sounding additives and chemicals, steer clear. Your best bet is to shop in a natural food store for condiments, where you'll find the healthiest selection.

streets of Florence, soaked in the history and architecture of Rome, and danced the flamenco in Barcelona. We made so many memories those 2 weeks that we'll never forget!

Travel takes you outside your normal day-to-day, which—let's face it—we can all use a break from now and then. It reminds you of what you love, what you're good at (who knew Karena was so good with a map?), and what inspires you.

So pack your bags, gorgeous. We're going on a road trip!

Your BE FIERCE Challenge:
Hit the Road

On Day 7 we challenged you to do a little exploring on your own. Today we're going to up the ante and challenge you to strike out (alone or with someone else) and do something new and different. Break new ground; test out the unknown; give something entirely unfamiliar a try. It doesn't matter what it is, as long as it's something you've never done before or someplace you've never been. Go make some new memories, girlfriend!

BOMBSHELL BONUS
Make Fun a Habit

Frisky is forever! Look for opportunities today (and every day going forward) to do things that make you smile or laugh. One of the most enjoyable things for us is to have a bunch of friends over and make dinner. We just talk, hang out, and laugh, and those are some of our best times. Or we'll take a picnic to the Hollywood Bowl and sit under the stars listening to great music. We make sure that every day has some sparkle in it—now you will too!

Here are a few ideas to get your spirit of adventure going . . .

- Take a hike to the very top of a mountain (that you've never climbed before).
- Hop on a ferry and see where it goes.
- Get on a bike and go for an unplanned ride.
- Pack up some yummy food and go on a picnic.

I recently took a road trip to Big Sur with one of my friends from back home. It was totally chaotic—we had no idea where we were going, made wrong turns all the way, got boxed out of the campground we were going to, and ended up having to sleep in the car. But we just laughed the entire time, and that made it into a fabulously fun adventure.—Karena

- Get an array of exotic fruits from the market and have a tasting party. (If you've never tasted a persimmon or dragon fruit, today's the day!)

- Go horseback riding.

- Strap on skates and go for a spin.

- Visit a landmark or tourist destination in your city or town that you've never explored.

- Go apple picking (if they're in season).

- Hit a flea market.

Be Fabulous

Today's a day to be sassy . . . be saucy . . . be flirty. In other words, be FABULOUS!

Your BE FABULOUS Challenge: *Bring It, Baby!*

Time to have some fun with the bombshell bod and confidence you're rocking. Why not . . .

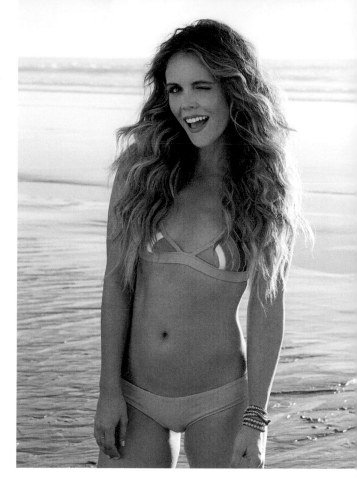

- Slide into some slinky heels.

- Ask your special someone to dance, right there at home. A slow dance in the living room or a morning twist-and-shout session while you're getting dressed is the best!

- Send a flirty text to someone you've had your eye on.

- Wear your sexiest bra today, even if no one will see it. (We know you've got one hidden in the drawer, and if not, go treat yourself to one!)

- Toss aside the after-work sweats and put on your good robe.

- Wink at a stranger (but be safe about it!).

- Rock a bewitching cat-eye with a flick of black gel eyeliner.

- Strut your stuff! Shoulders back. Smile on. Sashay like you're a superstar gracing the runway of life—because that's just what you are!

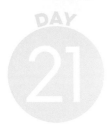

DAY

21

Sunday

Your Word for Today: Loving
Your Mantra: I am loved and have so much love to give.

Ohhhh . . . love. Sigh. So much we could say about love, but we want you to feel it, not read about it! So let's get you into a loving state of mind to launch you into your day of adoration and devotion.

Be Fit

Here is your BE FIT plan for today:

* Morning Booty Call
* Daily Fitness Challenge:
  Active rest day
* Fab Food of the Day:
  Sweet potatoes
* Body-Loving Recipe of the Day:
  Maple-Glazed Sweet Potatoes

Your Morning Booty Call

Love is the ultimate positive emotion. Today let it infuse every action you take, every word you say, and every thought you think—especially toward yourself. Open your heart and let in how worthy you are of admiration and adoration. And with that full, open heart, let your beautiful light shine out into the world.

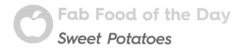

Fab Food of the Day
Sweet Potatoes

Seems perfectly right to feature a food today that's especially good for your ever-lovin' heart! Sweet potatoes—besides being divinely delish—are high in potassium, which helps lower blood pressure, and high in fiber, which lowers the risk of heart disease.

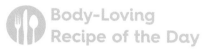

Body-Loving Recipe of the Day
Maple-Glazed Sweet Potatoes

Talk about loving: This recipe is a surefire way to a man's heart! This sweet, delicious dish is Karena's boyfriend Bobby's favorite; he grins ear to ear every time she whips it up for him.

Serves 2

- 1 pound sweet potatoes, chopped into squares
- 2 tablespoons extra-virgin olive oil
- 2 tablespoons pure maple syrup
- Sea salt, to taste
- 5 leaves fresh sage
- $1\frac{1}{2}$ tablespoons chopped fresh rosemary

Preheat the oven to 400°F.

On a cookie sheet or in a dish, place the sweet potatoes. Pour the oil, maple syrup, and salt on top and mix together with your hands. Top with the sage and rosemary. Bake for 40 to 50 minutes, or until the sweet potatoes are tender on the inside and crispy on the outside.

How do you love up your family and friends?

✳ I truly love finding something for someone that I feel they will really like. I'm on the lookout all year round for holiday and birthday gifts! I work hard for my paycheck, and when it comes down to it, I want to spend it on things that make me and the people I love happy!—Kate R.

✳ I love documenting fun memories with my family and friends in photos and posting them on Instagram.—Whitney M.

✳ I'm a fan of the random text message, just letting them know what you're up to and that you're thinking of them.—Katy L.

✳ I love to make goodies and gifts. I enjoy painting on canvas, making friendship bracelets (you're never too cool for friendship bracelets), and making them TIU-approved treats. I believe that a home-cooked meal is a gift from the heart.—Jenny N.

✳ My favorite way to express my love for my family and friends is just by being there for them no matter what.—Tiffany M.

Be Fierce

When life gets challenging, it's so tempting to be crabby, cynical, or angry. But you're here to grow fierce, and one of the best ways to do that is to staunchly say *NO WAY* to that negativity tornado. How do you resist it? Through the awe-inspiring power of L-O-V-E.

Like generosity and forgiveness, love expands you and crowds out everything else. When you're coming from a place of love, there is no room for negativity, or fear, or anger. Like we (and Karena's dad) said earlier, love always wins in the end. Love inspires and protects us. Today we want you to throw the doors to your heart open wide and just live from love.

Your BE FIERCE Challenge:
Turn On Your Love Lights

How can you express love? Let us count the ways! Choose one or more of these sweet karmic kisses . . .

- Write and send a genuine, old-school love letter to someone special in your life.

- Send a family member flowers—especially if they're not expecting it.

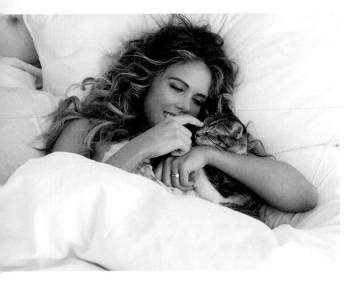

BOMBSHELL BONUS
Let Love In

Remember on Day 9, when we challenged you to say yes to offers and opportunities that came your way? Well, today we're upping the ante and asking you to say yes to acts of love. Let down your guard today and let the people who love you give from their hearts. Accept their hugs and their other gestures of adoration. Do it for them as a way to express your own love—and do it for you, who deserves buckets of love!

- Drop off a little gift for your Bombshell Buddy.

- Take your dog for a long walk, or give your kitty some bonus cuddles and ear rubs. Pets appreciate a little extra lovin' too!

- Bake a TIU-approved treat for your neighbor.

- Make your BFF's favorite dinner and invite her over.

- Give someone a hug (just make sure it's someone you know who is receptive to it!).

Be Fabulous

What do you say to a little pampering to make those pretty hands of yours all the more heavenly to hold? They do so much for you every day—type those brilliant e-mails, anchor your pushups, lift utensils, style your hair—so let's show them a little love in return.

Your BE FABULOUS Challenge:
Create a Marvelous Manicure

Start with this deliciously scented sweet-and-salty scrub. You'll need:

- 1 cup brown sugar
- 1 cup sea salt
- ¾ cup coconut oil
- 1 tablespoon extra-virgin olive oil
- 1 tablespoon vanilla extract
- 2 tablespoons lemon juice

In a medium bowl, mix together all of the ingredients. If needed, add another teaspoon or two of olive oil. (Tip: Keep the extra in a mason jar so you can give yourself a little pick-me-up next weekend too.)

Apply the mixture to your hands and scrub them gently to smooth and soften. Spend about 5 minutes massaging each hand. Give some extra attention to the pressure point between the thumb and index finger to promote tranquility (also great to relieve headaches and neck and upper back pain).

Rinse off the scrub and pat your hands dry. Next, prep your nails. Polish goes on and stays on best when nails are moisturized and

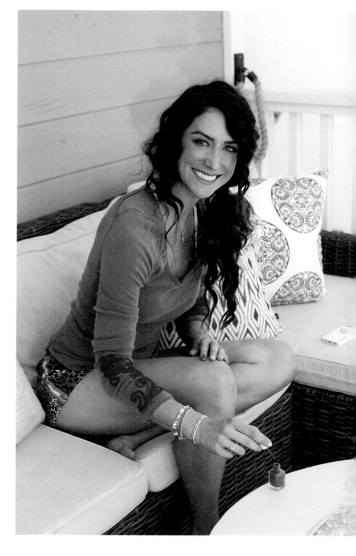

smooth. So grab a high-quality file and shape the edges; with a buffer, make the surfaces smooth. If you like, you can also push your cuticles back with an orange stick (most manicure kits you buy at the drugstore will have all the utensils you need).

Apply a high-quality base coat so your polish has something to adhere to, then apply a cute, fun color. Finish the job with a shiny topcoat to make your manicure last.

Don't forget to make this pampering experience fun! You could . . .

- Light a scented candle.
- Do it somewhere relaxing, like on your patio while the sun is setting.
- Pour yourself a little champagne and bring a magazine with you before you start so you can sip and read while your nails dry (and so you're not tempted to move around while they do!).
- Use nail art like glitter, jewels, or stickers for added flair.
- Pick a polish color that will coordinate with your outfit the next day.
- Invite your girlfriends over and have a manicure party.

End your day of love with a smile, knowing you cared for your beautiful self and made the world a little bit more of a loving place today with your presence.

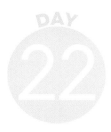

Monday

Your Word for Today: Energized
Your Mantra: Go, baby, go!

Sure, coffee is a great pick-me-up. But there are lots of other ways to get an energy blast! Today we're going to share our favorite (noncaffeinated) secrets to keep you revved up and rarin' to go.

Be Fit

Here is your BE FIT plan for today:

* Take and record your measurements.
* Morning Booty Call
* Daily Fitness Challenge:
  HIIT: HIIT the High Note (page 235)
* Fab Food of the Day:
  Spirulina
* Body-Loving Recipe of the Day:
  Spirulina Hummus

Take and Record Your Measurements

By this point, we're betting you're looking forward to whipping out that tape measure and seeing how much your body has transformed. As you should be! Repeat your measure-and-record process today and be sure to share the results at #FitFierceFab.

⏱ Your Morning Booty Call

We've got a treat to start off your day with some fab fun! Skip ahead and take the BE FIERCE challenge explained on the opposite page first thing in the morning.

We won't give away the surprise just yet, but let's put it this way: It'll get your heart pumping; put a big, bubbly bounce in your step; and fire up your energy for the whole day!

🍎 Fab Food of the Day
Spirulina

For a blast of nutritional energy, spirulina takes the top prize. This blue-green algae contains a whopping 4 to 8 grams of protein in just a 2-tablespoon serving! Spirulina is sold in a powder form, which makes it easy to add to your green juice or smoothies.

🍴 Body-Loving Recipe of the Day
Spirulina Hummus

Enjoy this garlicky, delicious, homemade hummus with sliced veggies or whole wheat pita slices.

Serves 2

- ½ 15-ounce can chickpeas, rinsed and drained
- ¼ cup tahini
- 3 tablespoons water
- 2 tablespoons fresh lemon juice

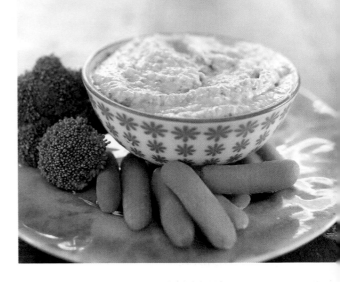

- 1 tablespoon spirulina
- 1 clove garlic, minced
- 1 tablespoon smoked paprika
- ½ teaspoon sea salt

In a food processor, blend together all ingredients until creamy.

Be Fierce

Sometimes a girl's just gotta dance. You know what we're saying, sisters?

We love, love, LOVE to dance! It's just so freeing. We have dance parties at our houses with our friends, blasting music and getting lost in it. Not long ago, we were away on an island teaching a retreat, and every night we stayed up until 4 a.m. dancing with a whole crew of Fit, Fierce, and Fabulous gals we'd just met. We danced and danced and danced. Not only was it crazy fun—it was the best workout ever!

Since then, we've made this kind of a Tone

Kat is an amazing dancer. She has such rhythm. I do not, but that doesn't stop me! I like to goof around and do my own version of "interpretive dancing." It usually ends up cracking us both up, and that only adds more to the fun.—Karena

It Up tradition. At our retreat in Newport Beach, hundreds of women danced in big groups every night, laughing and cheering each other on. You could tell everyone was having such a blast letting themselves dance wild and free like that. Sometimes even at the office, when a kick-ass song comes on, we'll get up and just start bopping around to the beat. It's an incredible way to get the energy going. Do we look silly? Maybe! But do we care? Heck, no!

Today we dare *you* to get movin' and groovin' and let your fierce flag fly!

Your BE FIERCE Challenge:
Shake It!

It doesn't matter if you turn on some tunes at home and dance by yourself or grab a partner and go out on the town to boogie down. Your mission for today is just to shake and shimmy that bombshell booty with abandon. Be wild. Be bold. Be free!

You're Invited to a Fierce, Fab Fiesta!

WHAT: A booty-shakin', soul-quakin', joy-makin' dance party

WHEN: Today

WHERE: Anywhere! (we like our living rooms, personally)

WHO: Beautiful you!

WHY: Why not?!

Be Fabulous

As if dancing wasn't already the absolute in energy blasts, there's more!

You already know from Day 12 how much aromas can calm and soothe you, but did you also know they can revitalize you with just one lusciously scented whiff?

When I hear music, I just feel like I need to move! I've never taken lessons, learned a routine, or danced professionally, but I think that's why I love it so much. It's still mine.—Katrina

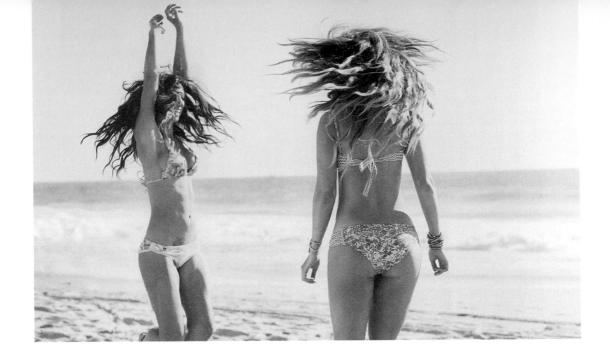

Your BE FABULOUS Challenge:
Revitalize with Scent

Here are the scents we love to use whenever we need a hit of invigorating energy:

- **Eucalyptus:** Put a dab on your wrists or use a spritzer before you get in the shower to make your own invigorating steam room. If you have a stuffy head, eucalyptus works wonders to clear it.

- **Lemon:** Lovely lemon is refreshing and detoxifying. Throughout the day, when you squeeze lemon into your water (which we know you're doing!), take a second or two to inhale its sweet scent. You can also mix a little lemon oil into your body lotion for an all-day lift.

- **Orange:** Orange helps increase mental focus. You can use orange oil, light a tangerine-scented candle, or simply peel an orange and leave the rinds on your desk to empower that sexy brain of yours.

- **Grapefruit:** This zingy citrus scent fights fatigue and is a known jet-lag cure.

- **Peppermint:** Make yourself a cup of peppermint tea for an instant mood lift. Peppermint is also great for increasing concentration and easing headaches.

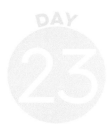
DAY
23

Tuesday

Your Word for Today: Authentic
Your Mantra: Today I will speak my mind.

Today is all about being true to *you*. What's on your mind? What are the truths in your heart? Today, with all our love and support, we're urging you to come out of hiding and fully reveal the Fit, Fierce, and Fabulous babe that you are.

Be Fit

Here is your BE FIT plan for today:

* Morning Booty Call
* Daily Fitness Challenge:
  Your choice
* Fab Food of the Day:
  Your choice
* Body-Loving Recipe of the Day:
  Your choice

Your Morning Booty Call

What feels right for you today? All day today, we want *you* to decide what resonates and works best for you. As long as you do both workouts (Booty Call and any one of the four Daily Fitness Challenges you've been doing), it's up to you what you do. *You* get to choose your superfood and recipe today. You've come a long way these past 3 weeks, and you're tuned in to your body and mind enough to know what will give you what you need.

BOMBSHELL BONUS
Honor Your Instincts

Deep down, you know what is right for you. Staying true to that is sometimes the challenge. Over the years, as we've built our Tone It Up brand, we've had offers and opportunities come our way that have been really lucrative and exciting but that weren't aligned with who we are and what we stand for. Some were really tempting to jump at, believe us! But ultimately we resisted, because we've learned that nothing is worth it if we're not being true to ourselves.

If something glittery comes along that you're unsure about—a job, a guy, an opportunity, even a purchase you're about to make—take a step back and give yourself time to think it over. Ask yourself, "Is this right for me?" Your heart will guide you in the right direction if you listen to its wisdom.

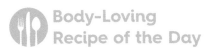

Fab Food of the Day

You choose! Which superfood so far has been your favorite? You can repeat the recipe listed for that food, come up with a new one on your own, or go to ToneItUp.com for other ideas.

Body-Loving Recipe of the Day

See above. Today you choose! Make something that fits your day and tantalizes your taste buds.

Be Fierce

Be honest: How often do you hold back what you're really thinking or keep quiet when there's something you need or want? It's so much easier to stay silent, but taking the easy path no longer suits a fierce fox like you. It's doing you no good to hush up—in fact, it's chipping away at the confidence and inner strength you've been cultivating.

Today your call to action is to be BOLD and speak your mind!

Your BE FIERCE Challenge:
Just Say It

Anytime you find yourself swallowing your opinion or needs today, out with it. The key is to speak your mind with kindness and respect, without apologizing. If you think something a coworker says is incorrect, tell him or her—respectfully. If your friends plan a dinner at a restaurant where you once got food poisoning and you can't bear to think of returning there, tell them—simply and directly—and suggest an alternative. You'll be amazed by how people respond. When you come from an authentic and honest stance, you'll find that people tend to relate to you more that way, and you'll feel a huge sense of relief by airing your truths.

By the way, this goes for the little things too. If a waiter forgot to put the dressing on the side of your salad, let him know. If the taxi driver is talking on the phone while he's

BOMBSHELL BONUS
Tackle the Tough Stuff

Is there one truth that's been gnawing at you? Something that's been hard to say, so you've avoided it? We've all been there. The problem with heavyweight secrets like these is that keeping them hidden sucks up all our good energy. If the time feels right, call upon your daringness and reach out to the person you need to talk to. More often than not, they won't be surprised by what you have to say, and you'll experience a breakthrough in your relationship one way or another that will set you both free.

driving and it makes you uncomfortable, politely ask him to hang up and continue his call later. Really, it's okay. You're allowed to have an opinion and make reasonable requests in this world.

Be Fabulous

No hiding today . . . and that means on the surface too! We want you to show the world your beautiful, real self.

Your BE FABULOUS Challenge: *Go Au Naturel*

Liberate yourself from makeup today. We know that might sound scary, since so many of us get dependent on our beauty products to make us feel beautiful. But with your new practices of eating lean, clean, and green foods; hydrating; sweating out toxins daily; using face masks; and relaxing and rejuvenating, your skin has no doubt got a FABULOUS glow. So put down the blush brush and let that beautiful, natural, authentic light shine today! (*Note:* If it's truly not possible for you to go bare-faced today because of an event or work, then choose at least an hour or two when you'll be out in public and can do this.)

I wear my heart on my sleeve; it's hard for me to hide anything, so if something's bothering me, you'll hear about it. It's good because there's no surprise later, and things always improve because we have something to work on. I think communicating openly with others is the best way to grow as a person, as a couple, or as a friend.—Katrina

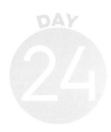

Wednesday

Your Word for Today: Strong
Your Mantra: I am mighty. I am strong. I am FIERCE!

Buckle up, superwoman—you're about to surprise yourself! You're a force to be reckoned with, and today we're going to prove it. Wait . . . scratch that. Today you're going to prove it to yourself.

Be Fit

Here is your BE FIT plan for today:

* Morning Booty Call
* Daily Fitness Challenge:
  Full-Body Toning: Rock It Like You
  Mean It (page 209)
* Fab Food of the Day:
  Quinoa
* Body-Loving Recipe of the Day:
  Baked Quinoa-Stuffed Tomato

Your Morning Booty Call

This is a great day to sculpt those gorgeous muscles with some extra strength training. Blast off your day with the Amazing Abs and Arms (page 247), Booty Shorts (page 251), or Burn, Baby, Burn (page 214) HIIT workout and feel your body growing stronger with every stretch, curl, lift, and lunge.

Fab Food of the Day
Quinoa

Quinoa is one of our favorite foods because it's a complete protein that provides you with all the essential amino acids your gorgeous, strong body needs. It's a seed, but it cooks up just like a grain. Quinoa has it all: It's gluten-free, low glycemic (so it won't spike your blood sugar), rich in iron to keep your blood cells healthy, and packed with magnesium, manganese, and vitamin B_2, which boost energy and metabolism and improve brain and muscle function. So go ahead and power up your day with this potent protein!

Body-Loving Recipe of the Day
Baked Quinoa-Stuffed Tomato

With its mild, nutty flavor, quinoa makes this recipe a savory surprise hit at any gathering.

Serves 2

- 2 large ripe tomatoes
- Sea salt and pepper, to taste
- 1 cup water
- ½ cup quinoa
- 2 teaspoons grape seed oil
- ¼ yellow onion, chopped
- 2 cloves garlic, chopped

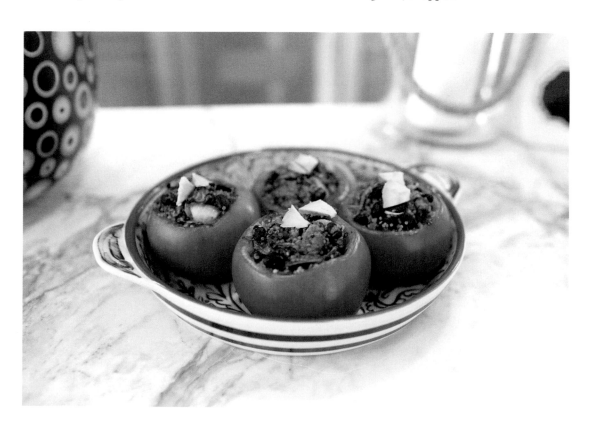

- ½ cup black beans (freshly cooked or, if canned, rinsed)
- 2 cups fresh baby spinach
- Few slices avocado (optional)

Preheat the oven to 375°F.

Destem and hollow out the tomatoes. Sprinkle a pinch of salt and pepper inside each and place in a flat baking dish.

In a saucepan, combine the water and quinoa and bring to a boil. Lower to a simmer for 10 to 15 minutes, or until the quinoa is fully cooked.

In a separate saucepan, heat the oil on low and sauté the onion and garlic for 5 minutes. Add the black beans, spinach, and a pinch more salt and pepper and stir until the spinach is wilted. Add the cooked quinoa from the other saucepan and stir everything together.

Scoop the quinoa mixture and stuff it into the tomatoes. Bake for 15 to 20 minutes, or until the tomato starts to soften and the quinoa turns golden brown. We like to top these with a few slices of avocado for garnish.

Be Fierce

You already know Karena's very personal triathlon story, which shows how powering your way through something challenging can inspire some pretty fierce warrior spirit (it's back on page 3, if you want a reminder). Don't worry—we're not going to insist you do a triathlon today (but don't rule it out for sometime soon!). You're going to do something else that strengthens that inner reserve in a slightly quieter—but no less powerful—way.

Your BE FIERCE Challenge:
Take a Bad Habit Holiday

What's your worst habit? Do you bite your nails? Procrastinate? Neglect to call people back? Are you quick to be snippy with your sweetie? C'mon, fess up. We all have at least one!

We know these habits can be tough to break; we're right there with you. So we're going to start small. Just like building up muscle, building willpower comes from starting with something just a little challenging, then a

We'll admit it: We're both chronically late. It's something we're trying to work on, so we've been making a super-conscious effort lately to be on time for everything—we are really improving! It's not easy, but we feel so good when we pull it off. xo K&K

BOMBSHELL BONUS
Declare Every Wednesday "Bad Habit–Free Hump Day"

Ready for a little more inner strength building? Continue your one-day-at-a-time bad habit break by repeating it every Wednesday. Trust us, you'll wake up on Thursdays feeling like a total rock star!

little more, then a little more. Before you know it, you're a tower of strength and stamina.

So for now, forget trying to give up this habit forever. That would be like running a marathon without training. We want to make this realistic and doable, so just for today, make a deliberate effort to shelve this habit. Call back each person who reaches out to you. Show up on time. Tackle that pile of paperwork that's been lingering. We're talking roughly 15 hours from the time you wake up until the time you go to bed—that's a teeny-tiny commitment for someone as fierce as you. Prove to yourself that you can do it! The point is to build the strength that comes from conviction. Maybe you're not ready to give it up all the time, but this is a great step in the right direction.

Be Fabulous

Sometimes it helps to have a visual reminder of just how mighty a force you really are. Karena has a tattoo on her wrist of the Japanese symbol for strength. Every time she catches a glimpse of it, it's a cue for her to be strong, no matter what comes her way. We're not suggesting you need to go out and get a tattoo; there are plenty of ways to symbolize your own inner strength.

Your BE FABULOUS Challenge:
Find Your Power Symbol

Take some time today to think about what represents strength for you and display it somewhere that you'll see it often. Here are just a few ideas:

- Put a photo on your desk of someone you admire who embodies strength.

- Wear a piece of jewelry that makes you feel grounded and in your power. Topaz and tigereye are two stones known to fortify strength, and hematite is wonderful for grounding.

- Write or paint a sign with empowering words and phrases on it.

- Release your inner wildcat! Lions are the most powerful animal in the jungle, so find an image of this mighty animal to inspire your inner fierceness.

What represents personal strength to you?

✳ My running shoes. When I started running 9 years ago, I couldn't even run 30 seconds straight because of my asthma; now I am running half- and full marathons. My lungs are so much stronger than they used to be!—Amy M.

✳ Anything and everything Tone It Up, from the famous wave heart to mermaids or seashells. —Chelsea S.

✳ I got my first mala beads from my husband as a wedding gift and I love wearing them. Whenever I wear/touch/am around them, I truly do feel more connected to inspiration, creativity, acceptance, and love. If I know I'm going to have a tough day or will need some extra strength, I make sure to put them on.—Kate R.

✳ A photo of my grandmother. She was an incredible woman, and every time I look at her picture, I'm reminded how much she believed in me. —Donna R.

✳ The Serenity Prayer helps guide me in acknowledging there are things I need to let go of and there are things I need to do differently. Accepting can be a difficult and uncomfortable challenge, but it takes personal strength to move forward.—Martha P.

✳ I wear a ring that has the quote "Though she be but little she is fierce" engraved on it.—Dina A.

✳ My mason jar keepsake from the Tone It Up retreat that I made. Inside of it you will find a piece of my yoga mat and some sand from the Booty Call I did on the beach with K&K. I did moves I never thought I'd be able to do—it was an extremely proud moment for me. —Candice M.

✳ The medal I got for running my first 5-K gives me strength to run the extra mile every time I look at it.—Debbie M.

● The scents of cedarwood, sage, and ylang-ylang are believed to fortify strength. If their scent has this effect for you, light a candle or use their essential oil in an aromatherapy bath.

● Wear a scarf in your power color. Red is typically the shade associated with strength, but for you, it might be vivid purple, deep blue, chocolate brown, or jet black.

Whatever works for you, use it to inspire you to be the powerhouse you are—not just today, but every day.

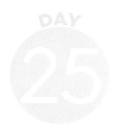

Thursday

Your Word for Today: Inspired
Your Mantra: Magic and wonder are all around me.

Turned on, lit up, psyched, filled with wonder . . . call it whatever you want—those are the juicy moments we live for!

Be Fit

Here is your BE FIT plan for today:

* Morning Booty Call
* Daily Fitness Challenge:
  HIIT: HIIT the High Note (page 235)
* Fab Food of the Day:
  Mint
* Body-Loving Recipe of the Day:
  Watermelon, Mint, and Arugula Salad

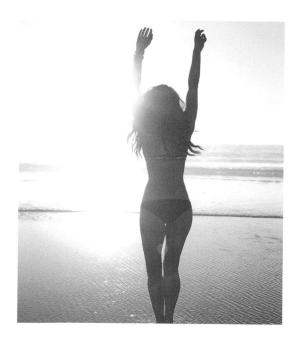

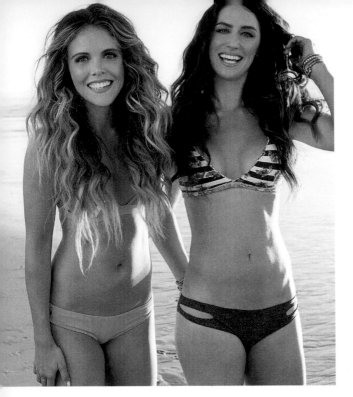

Fab Food of the Day
Mint

Today's a day for being exhilarated, and what's more invigorating than fresh mint? Mint contains tons of antioxidants and is even known as an appetite suppressant (the scent and flavor helps reduce cravings!).

Body-Loving Recipe of the Day
Watermelon, Mint, and Arugula Salad

We're California girls at heart, so for us, anything that screams summer—like this bright and refreshing salad—is a winner!

Serves 2

- ¾ cup high-quality balsamic vinegar
- 2 cups arugula
- 3 tablespoons chopped fresh mint
- 3 cups cubed watermelon
- ¼ cup feta cheese or crumbled tofu

In a saucepan, simmer the vinegar over medium heat for 6 to 7 minutes, or until it reduces to a maple syrup–like consistency. Remove from the heat and allow to cool.

Your Morning Booty Call

Today we have a special Booty Call suggestion for you. Set your alarm and wake up just before the sun. There's instant inspiration, right there in the sky! It's the perfect time to do some yin yoga (see page 257). As you breathe and stretch, let the early morning stillness infuse you with its quiet beauty. This day holds infinite potential—just like you.

Tantalizing Tip:

Next time you feel that 3 p.m. slump, give your brain a boost by brewing a cup of mint tea. The scent has been shown to increase alertness and productivity.

Combine the arugula, mint, watermelon, and cheese or tofu in a bowl. Mix and dress with the balsamic glaze immediately before serving.

Be Fierce

You might think inspiration is something that just hits you, almost by random happy luck. But just like fun and adventure, you can actually make it happen. No more waiting around for lightning to strike or your muse to mysteriously appear. Today you're going to spark up your life all by your fierce and fabulous self.

Your BE FIERCE Challenge:
Seek Out Your Sparkle

What do you love? What makes your toes curl, makes you feel bouncy and bubbly, or puts a twinkle in your eye? Where and when do you get your biggest and best ideas? Some of you may find inspiration being near the sea or riding your bike. For others it may come when you're listening to music, volunteering, or having a deep conversation with a fascinating person. If there's something you already know does it for you, make a concerted effort today to do it (or if it's something you need to plan, like a trip, then take the first steps to making that happen).

If you're not sure what lights you up, all

BOMBSHELL BONUS
Keep an Inspiration Inventory

Starting today, *bored* is no longer in your fierce vocabulary! Anytime you come across something that excites or moves you in a positive way, write it down. Keep a list somewhere accessible (on your phone, for instance) of all the things that make you feel happy and engaged. That way, anytime you are feeling blah or just want an added hit of inspiration, you'll have your options right there in front of you, ready to go.

the better, because today you're going to make some amazing discoveries! There are lots of ways to find what inspires you. Why don't you . . .

- Read a magazine or blog you've never read before.

- Explore an art gallery.

- Seek out something beautiful (seashells glittering in the sun, to-die-for dresses in a shop window, the smile of someone you love).

- Go to an exhibit at a museum that seems interesting to you.

- Listen to a type of music that you don't normally.

Where do you find inspiration?

✳ By the water. It doesn't have to be the beach, but it helps if there's sand in my toes. —Kate R.

✳ Hiking and exploring in Fundy National Park. It's about 45 minutes to an hour from my house and it is so beautiful there.—Amy M.

✳ I am most inspired when I see someone doing something good, in whatever capacity. It restores my faith in humankind.—Tiffany M.

✳ Browsing in a bookstore.—Ava G.

✳ Talking to my sister. She's the wisest, most fascinating person on the planet!—Donna R.

- Visit the oldest person you know (elderly people are filled with fascinating stories).

- Visit the youngest person you know (the clarity and innocence of babes can change your whole perspective).

- Sit outside a café and watch the people go by.

- Watch an uplifting movie. A good chick flick is always a great choice! Karena's favorite movie to watch over and over (and over . . .) again is *The Holiday*. Kat loves *The Sweetest Thing*, and our number-one favorite for joint movie night is *It's Complicated*.

- Try a restaurant, dish, or recipe that's intriguing to you.

- Ask your friends to show you their favorite thing or place. What they've already discovered might be just what you're looking for!

The trick is to watch for that little flicker when something catches your eye or nudges your interest. When you feel it, grab hold of the opportunity and go with it! That little electric jolt is the seed of inspiration; all it needs is your attention and willingness to bloom.

Be Fabulous

Now that you've got your inspiration lights shining, let's keep that going with one of Karena's favorite imagination igniters: a fabulous book!

Reading is relaxing, but there's more to it than just that. Reading helps you grow by learning about yourself and seeing thing from a different perspective. Just like dancing (which, as you already know, is number one on Kat's list of inspiring activities), reading transports you. As you get absorbed in the story, you're fully present and your mind expands as it takes in the beauty of good writing. Tonight we offer you this challenge to cap off your inspired day.

Your BE FABULOUS Challenge:
Fire Up Your Imagination

Already have a book going? Great! If not, choose one you've been meaning to get around

BOMBSHELL BONUS
Book a Buddy

We're now doing our own private little book club. It's so much fun to hear each other's perspectives on what we read! Reading a book along with someone else changes up the conversation and lets you grow together. Tomorrow when you meet up with your Bombshell Buddy, why not suggest that you and she read an inspiring book together?

to reading. If it's not already on your bookshelf, pick up a copy of it sometime today, download it, or borrow it from a friend or the library (yes, there are still libraries, and they're often the best-kept secret around). And if you don't have a book in mind, ask your friends for a suggestion or just take a browse through your local bookstore or look online. Fiction or nonfiction, there is no shortage of incredible reads out there.

Start your evening routine a little earlier tonight and aim to read one full chapter. Getting lost in a good book even for a few minutes will open your mind in astonishing ways.

I read a ton of nonfiction. *Tuesdays with Morrie* is a book I've read like five times and give to people as a gift all the time.—Karena

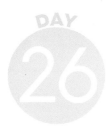

DAY

26

Friday

Your Word for Today: Radiant
Your Mantra: I am a glowing beam of love and joy.

Look at that gorgeous glow you've got going! You've done so many body-nourishing, soul-deepening, heart-opening things since starting this program, and today we want to make sure to capture them all to keep you radiating forever.

Be Fit

Here is your BE FIT plan for today:

* Morning Booty Call

* Daily Fitness Challenge:
  Active rest day

* Fab Food of the Day:
  Flaxseeds

* Body-Loving Recipe of the Day:
  Tropical Green Smoothie

Your Morning Booty Call

It's a rest day, so with your lighter Booty Call, you probably have a little extra time this morning. Perfect opportunity to do a morning meditation! See page 66 for a review of how to meditate and awaken your inner radiance.

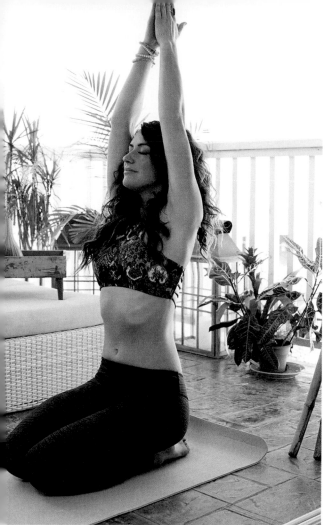

to give that smooth, beautiful skin of yours even more radiance.

Body-Loving Recipe of the Day
Tropical Green Smoothie

Transport your mind to an island getaway as you supercharge your day and fuel your body with the nutrients it needs for glowing, dewy skin!

Serves 2

- 2 cups fresh spinach
- $\frac{1}{2}$ cup frozen peaches
- $\frac{1}{2}$ cup frozen pineapple
- $\frac{1}{2}$ cup frozen mango
- $\frac{1}{2}$ cup coconut water
- $\frac{1}{2}$ cup unsweetened almond milk
- 1 tablespoon flaxseed meal
- 2 tablespoons unsweetened shredded coconut

In a blender, process all ingredients except the coconut until smooth. Top with the coconut before serving.

Fab Food of the Day
Flaxseeds

Foods loaded with omega-3s are a beauty gold mine, and flaxseeds are no exception. We're including them as today's Fab Food of the Day

Tantalizing Tip

Grind whole flaxseeds in a coffee grinder and use the flax meal to thicken sauces and salad dressings.

Be Fierce

Everything you've been doing up until now in your BE FIERCE challenges has been to empower your inner tigress. She's sleek. She's strong. She moves with the sexy assuredness of someone who knows who she is and what she wants. And while she herself cannot be caged, today she is going to corral all the positive actions that make her the dynamic, awe-inspiring creature she is.

Your BE FIERCE Challenge:
Revel, Record, Radiate

Take some time today to review all the positive practices you've done over the past 26 days. Read through this list below—you've actually accomplished all these things! The goal here is to identify the challenges that had the most impact on you, because those are the ones you'll want to be sure to continue.

Since Day 1 you've:

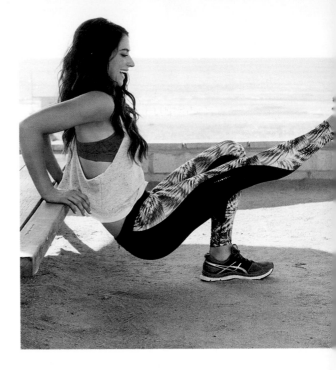

- Committed to your goals
- Motivated yourself with your vision boar
- Created a morning ritual
- Nixed the negativity
- Set "I'm gorgeous!" reminders for yourself
- Ended your day with a gratitude list
- Gone on a solo adventure
- Done at least one thing that scared you
- Looked people in the eye
- Gotten your artistic groove on

I can always spot a Fit, Fierce, and Fabulous gal, because she has an unmistakable radiance. You can just tell that she knows deep down how lucky she is to be confident and healthy, and that she has the knowledge and tools to take care of herself. Just like you!—Karena

Shine On, Sunshine!

That question about which practices lit you up inside and which you'll commit to wasn't rhetorical—we really want to know! Post your list to #FitFierceFab to share the love and inspire your Fit, Fierce, and Fabulous sisters, just as they have inspired you.

- Put yourself first with your list of daily nonnegotiables
- Reflected on and recorded your progress in your journal
- Decluttered your space
- Taken one day to simply *chill*
- Tuned in to each present moment
- Practiced being selfless
- Learned to accept what comes your way
- Opened your heart to forgive and show your love
- Sung your heart out and danced with abandon!
- Done something spontaneous or out of your usual routine
- Bravely spoken your mind

- Taken a break from a bad habit
- Invited inspiration

What BE FIERCE practices filled you most with love, pride, and joy? Which ones will you commit to going forward? Write them in your journal as a promise to yourself. You've already tapped into the power of self-commitment—now use it to fuel your Fit, Fierce, and Fabulous life!

Be Fabulous

You're already glowing on the inside . . . so let's get you glimmering, shimmering skin on the outside to match! Today we'll share our top tips and pointers for getting that bronzy, bombshell glow.

Your BE FABULOUS Challenge:
Get the Eternal Sunshine Shimmer

Here's all you need to know to look sultry and summer-kissed, without forgoing the all-important SPF (remember, always use sunscreen under your makeup, even if you think you don't need it!):

- Always start with soft, smooth skin. Coconut oil is our *miracle* for face and body. It leaves you feeling silky, and the smell is heavenly.

- Exfoliate a few times per week to slough off dulling dead skin. Use a natural product from the store or make your own (see page 113).

- For a bright complexion, use a tinted moisturizer and illuminator. We like Laura Mercier Tinted Moisturizer and VS PRO Radiant FX Face Illuminator. Remember to smooth it on lightly—more isn't necessarily better.

- If you want to dial down the shimmer, use a matte bronzer like Marc Jacobs O!Mega Bronze.

- If you want to do some sunless tanner, don't forget to use plastic gloves (tan palms are a dead giveaway!), and make sure not to put too much in the creases of your ankles, elbows, and knees. We want sexy, not stripy!

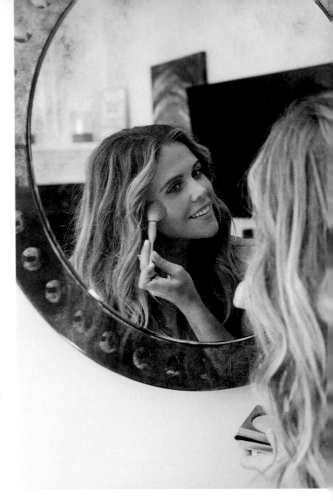

- Dab a little illuminator directly under your eyes to lighten and brighten. A touch also looks beautiful on your collarbones or on the peaks of your shoulders.

- One of the best tips we got from our makeup artist for daytime is to forgo glittery eye shadows and go with a more subtle palate of shimmery cream, gold, bronze, cocoa, and soft rose. The effect is pretty magical.

- A pink or red cheek stain is an instant way to get a fresh, rosy glow.

- Hydrate, hydrate, hydrate! Keep drinking all that H_2O and you'll have healthy, vibrant skin that radiates all on its own.

- Don't forget the ultimate bombshell secret: SMILE! Flash those pearly whites and you're guaranteed to dazzle.

I always say that the most beautiful curve on a woman's body is her smile.—Katrina

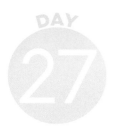
DAY

Saturday

Dear Amazing You,

You're almost at the end of your Fit, Fierce, and Fabulous launch. You've worked so hard over the past 4 weeks, and you deserve to really take it in.

You woke up for more Booty Calls than you ever imagined you could, made healthy decisions, tried new things, drank gallons of fresh water, and (we hope!) made inspiring new girlfriends through the Tone It Up community. You ate tons of greens—and actually started craving them! You held strong to your commitments to yourself, took the stairs when you could have cruised, and resisted the temptation of excess sweets because you know your life will be so much sweeter for it.

Best of all, you did it all willingly, with an open heart. You may have secretly cussed at us when your alarm went off first thing in the morning, or screamed and grunted at us during some of your workouts, but you did it. YOU DID IT! Whether you reached big or small goals, met milestones, or just realized how to communicate with your body and live boldly, your dedication to your well-being is pretty freaking amazing, and we just want to tell you we are so proud of you.

Let's all continue to be healthy, happy, and confident and treat ourselves with respect. From today on, every time you talk to yourself, do it with pride and gratitude. You're too fierce and fabulous now to be critical of yourself or of other women. You don't give yourself grief for setbacks or mistakes you make. You hiccup and bounce back even stronger! Every experience makes you wiser and better.

Promise yourself this right now: Every single day is going to be one to remember, because you're going to live them all to the fullest! When you're 80 and sitting with your grandchildren, you'll have pictures and stories to tell. You'll share with them how you were spontaneous, went on adventures, and met new people whom you still know today. You'll tell them your lifelong truth: Every day, we all have opportunities to live big and be our most fit, fierce, and fabulous self. They're ours for the taking.

xo, Karena and Katrina

Be Fit

Here is your BE FIT plan for today:

* Morning Booty Call
* Daily Fitness Challenge: Cardio: The Victory Lap (page 245)
* Fab Food of the Day: Garlic
* Body-Loving Recipe of the Day: Savory Turkey Burgers

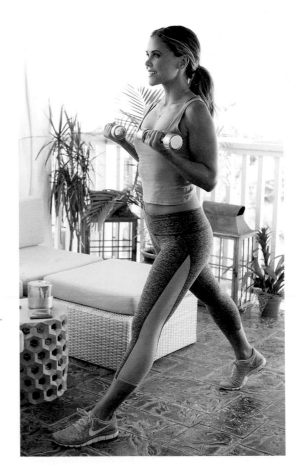

Your Morning Booty Call

This is your last Saturday with us guiding you, but really, you're ready to fly on your own. Today wake up and choose your Booty Call with all the confidence, motivation, and self-awareness that is now yours to keep.

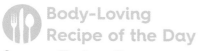

Fab Food of the Day
Garlic

This is Karena's favorite! Besides adding crazy-good flavor to dishes, garlic contains manganese, vitamin B_6, antioxidants, and valued sulfur compounds that keep your heart healthy.

Body-Loving Recipe of the Day
Savory Turkey Burgers

These bold and flavorful turkey burgers are always a hit at our neighborhood BBQs, and they're Katrina's hubby Brian's "happy meal"! He gets so excited when he hears these are on the menu.

Serves 2

- ½ pound 99% fat-free organic ground turkey
- ½ cup egg whites (or 4 egg whites)
- 3 tablespoons extra-virgin olive oil
- 3 tablespoons fat-free feta cheese
- 2 cloves garlic, minced
- ¼ cup chopped fresh spinach
- ¼ cup chopped fresh basil
- Pinch of thyme
- 2 cups green leafy lettuce

In a large bowl, mix together the ground turkey, egg whites, oil, feta, garlic, spinach, basil, and thyme. Form into 2 patties.

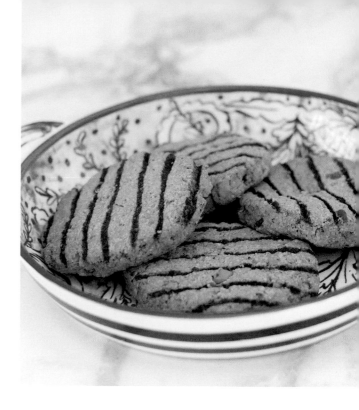

Heat the grill to medium and cook the patties for 8 minutes on each side, or until they reach an internal temperature of 165°F.

Serve each burger over a bed of lettuce or on a whole wheat bun.

Be Fierce

We know how much you've truly accomplished, but do *you*? We want you to not just know it, but OWN IT!

Your BE FIERCE Challenge:
Rack Up Your Victories

Take out your journal and get ready to be astonished by yourself. Here's what we challenge you to fill out:

Body

When I started this program, physically I felt: _____

Today I feel: _____

My energy at the beginning was at level (1–10): _____

Today it is at level: _____

On Day 1 my measurements were: _____

Today they are: _____

In the beginning I was able to run or walk this much/this far: _____

Today I can go: _____

The things I struggled with in the beginning but that now feel doable or easy are: _____

Mind

On Day 1 I felt these emotions: _____

Today I feel: _____

When I started this program, I had these doubts: _____

Today I believe I can: _____

In the beginning I prioritized my needs and self-care to this level (1–10): _____

Today I prioritize them to this level: _____

Before beginning this program, when faced with a challenge or struggle, I would: _____

Now I do this: _____

Spirit

In the spirit of love I have grown in these ways: _____

In the spirit of generosity I have expanded in these ways: _____

In the spirit of joy I have changed my outlook in these ways: _____

In the spirit of beauty and radiance I now see myself in this glorious light: _____

Pretty amazing, isn't it? Now it's not just us who are proud of you. It's you who is very deservedly applauding yourself.

Be Fabulous

We don't know about you, but to us, hard work calls for a reward!

Your BE FABULOUS Challenge:
Reward Yourself

If we were there with you in person, we'd be giving you a great big present right about now. But since we're not, we're going to have to trust you to do it for us.

What's the one thing that you can give yourself that will forever remind you of your Fit, Fierce, and Fabulous victories? It can be a thing, like a new outfit; a workout video or class pack; a spiffy new pair of sneaks; a piece of jewelry; or a beautiful new journal to keep your fierce new practice going. Or it can be an experience, a retreat, a visit somewhere you've been wanting to go, or a special meal with your Bombshell Buddies to celebrate your accomplishments.

Whatever it is, your only mandate for today is to enjoy it. You've earned it!!

What's your favorite way to reward yourself?

✳ I love treating myself to a massage, a manicure, or a facial.—Stephanie F.

✳ Air-popped popcorn, dark chocolate, and Tone It Up gear.—Krystie S.

✳ Workout clothes! Is there anything better? It also gets me excited to go work out so that I can wear my new gear!—Kelli R.

✳ A nice Epsom salt bath.—Amy M.

✳ Definitely chocolate (just one square of dark chocolate, I swear!).—Katy L.

✳ If I'm feeling saucy, I'll reward myself with a new dress. Clothing is a great treat.—Jenny N.

✳ A fun night out!—Divya R.

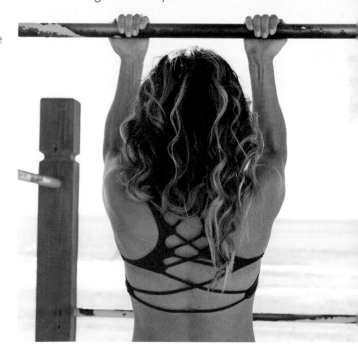

What are you proud of?

✳ I am proud of myself for making the effort to take care of my body and encouraging my kids to do the same by eating clean and working out with me.—Kelli R.

✳ Exercise is now something I do to protect, love, and care for my body—not to change it because I hate it.—Tiffany M.

✳ I've had multiple setbacks in my journey from health, both physical and emotional. I've been able to find that strength within to keep going. No matter how many times I get knocked down, I keep fighting to reach my goals.—Candice M.

✳ All through high school and college, I shamed my body: my booty was too big, my hips too wide, my hair too curly . . . I could go on and on. I would never accept a compliment. But now, I LOVE my body. I love my big booty, I love my curves, I love my wild hair, my smile. Tone It Up helped me recognize that I am strong and beautiful inside and out.—Jenny N.

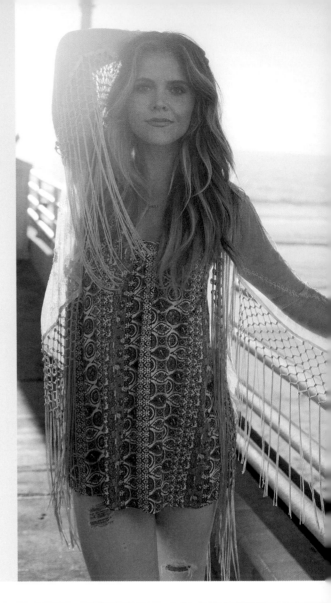

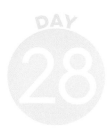

DAY

28

Sunday

This is it . . . you made it! Congratulations for all you've accomplished. You are a Fit, Fierce, and Fabulous tour de force! From here, all that's left to conquer is one question:

"What's next?"

Be Fit

Here is your BE FIT plan for today:

* Morning Booty Call

* Daily Fitness Challenge:
  Cardio: Rock It Like You Mean It
  (page 209)

* Fab Food of the Day:
  Brussels sprouts

* Body-Loving Recipe of the Day:
  Cheesy Buffalo Brussels Bites

Your Morning Booty Call

This morning as you toss off the covers for your Morning Booty Call, take a moment to reflect back to how you felt on that first day . . . and now look at you! You've worked hard to adopt a bona fide healthy lifestyle that is now yours to keep.

This is the perfect day to rock a heart-pumping HIIT Booty Call routine like HIIT and Run on page 254 or Firecracker Intervals on page 255. See how far you've come since Day 1!

Fab Food of the Day
Brussels Sprouts

Packed with everything from fiber to antioxidants to tons of vitamins and minerals, Brussels sprouts help fight harmful inflammation in the body, prevent disease and strengthen your bones. Roasted, shaved raw, or made into the irresistible party favorite below, we can't get enough of these delicious cruciferous crusaders!

Body-Loving Recipe of the Day
Cheesy Buffalo Brussels Bites

Cheesy, spicy, and every bit as satisfying as traditional hot wings, these are perfect for game day or a night in with friends. You may want to double the recipe—these little bites won't last long!

Serves 2

- 1½ cups low-sodium vegetable broth
- 1½ cups Brussels sprouts
- 1 tablespoon grape seed oil
- 1 teaspoon minced fresh garlic
- Sea salt, to taste
- 2 tablespoons hot buffalo sauce of your choice (most natural food stores have an array to choose from)
- ⅛ cup nutritional yeast
- ¼ teaspoon cayenne pepper

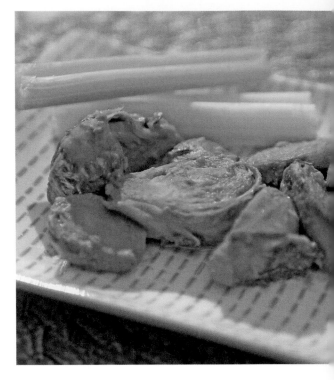

In a medium saucepan, bring the broth to a boil and add the Brussels sprouts. Allow to simmer for about 3 minutes, or until they turn bright green. Drain and rinse in cold water for 30 seconds before cutting each sprout in half.

Heat a sauté pan on medium and add the oil. When warm, add the garlic and salt and allow to simmer for 1 minute. Add the halved Brussels sprouts to the pan cut side down and sauté until brown, about 6 to 8 minutes.

Allow the sprouts to cool slightly before tossing with hot sauce, nutritional yeast, and cayenne pepper. Serve warm or cold and garnish with carrots and celery sticks!

Be Fierce

Today may be your last day of this program, but it's only the beginning of your remarkable journey. From here, anything is possible!

Your BE FIERCE Challenge:
Make Your Plan

What's next for you? What do you want to continue on to accomplish? What goals have you already begun dreaming about for yourself? Today we challenge you to make a written pact with yourself for the days to come. Once again, we want you to tap the incredible power of visualization! Take out your Fit, Fierce, and Fabulous Journal and write your answers to these questions:

- What are my next goals for my body?
- How, specifically, will I make those happen?
- What are my next goals for my overall state of mind?

- How will I make that happen?
- What are my goals for how I show up in the world and relate to others?
- How and when will I put that into practice?
- What do I want to accomplish in my work?
- How will I make that happen?
- What do I want to make happen in my personal life?
- How will I create that for myself?

With the answers to these questions in hand, we have one last BE FIERCE challenge for you: Use everything you've learned over the past 28 days and *go make it happen!*

Be Fabulous

Remember how on Day 26 you reviewed all your BE FIERCE challenges to see which

I'm a HUGE fan of Brussels sprouts. They were my enemy as a kid, but now I just can't get enough. They're full of antioxidants and vitamins like A, C, and E. For a quick dinner I will toss them in a cooking dish with a bit of olive oil, sea salt, pepper, cayenne, and cinnamon and bake at 450°F for 30 to 35 minutes.—Karena

ones had the most impact on you? Well, today we want you to do the same for your BE FABULOUS challenges, because dazzling from the inside counts every bit as much!

Over the past 28 days, you've:

- Made an "I'm Amazing" list
- Found (and been) a Bombshell Buddy
- Absorbed the calm influence of nature
- Taken "me time" for pampering and experimented with body scrubs, aromatherapy baths, and DIY face and hair masks
- Planned a date night with your bestie to express your love and gratitude
- Rocked a new color or hairstyle
- Had some fun mixing it up in your closet
- Joined up with other Fit, Fierce, and Fabulous gals
- Adopted some new beauty rituals to get soft, sultry lips, gorgeous hands and nails, and that unmistakable bombshell glow
- Done a tech detox
- Shared your culinary goodness
- Learned to accept your beautiful body just as it is
- Let the little annoyances slide
- Made your home a happy haven

BOMBSHELL BONUS
Be Loud and Proud!

Sound the trumpets—you're a warrior princess with a victory to proclaim! Don't forget to share your accomplishments with the Tone It Up community. Not only will you feel extra proud—you'll encourage and inspire others who are just beginning their journey. There's a Fit, Fierce, and Fabulous revolution happening, and you're a big part of it!

- Gotten a little frisky!
- Fired up your imagination with a good book
- Shared your accomplishments with the Tone It Up community
- Rewarded your remarkable self

Which were your favorites? Which will you commit to going forward, to keep yourself smiling and radiating each and every day? Shine on, sister!

A Final Word

This isn't good-bye . . . far from it! You're now an invaluable part of the Tone It Up commu-

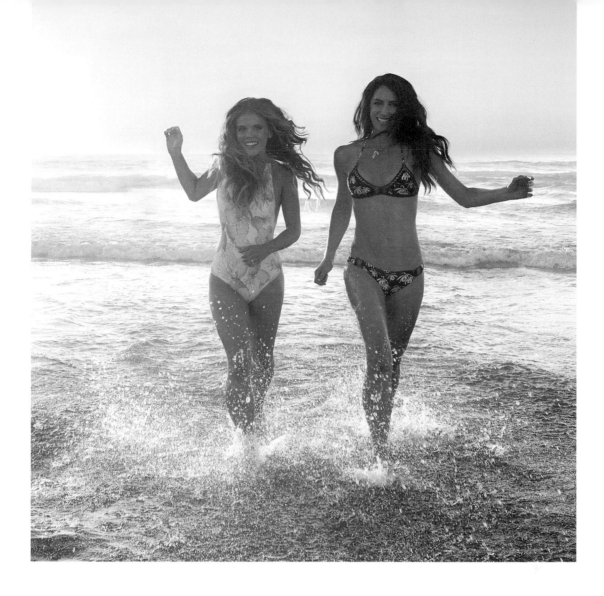

nity, and we—and your Fit, Fierce, and Fabulous sisters—want to see you continue with all the amazing lifestyle changes you've made. Check in and keep on sharing your accomplishments! We know, without a shadow of a doubt, that you're going to rock everything you do. We started this program telling you that we believe in you. And now we hope you believe in yourself—because you really *can* do anything you set that fierce and fabulous mind to. You've now got all the tools it takes to achieve anything you want for your body and in your life.

Remember, you are UNSTOPPABLE!

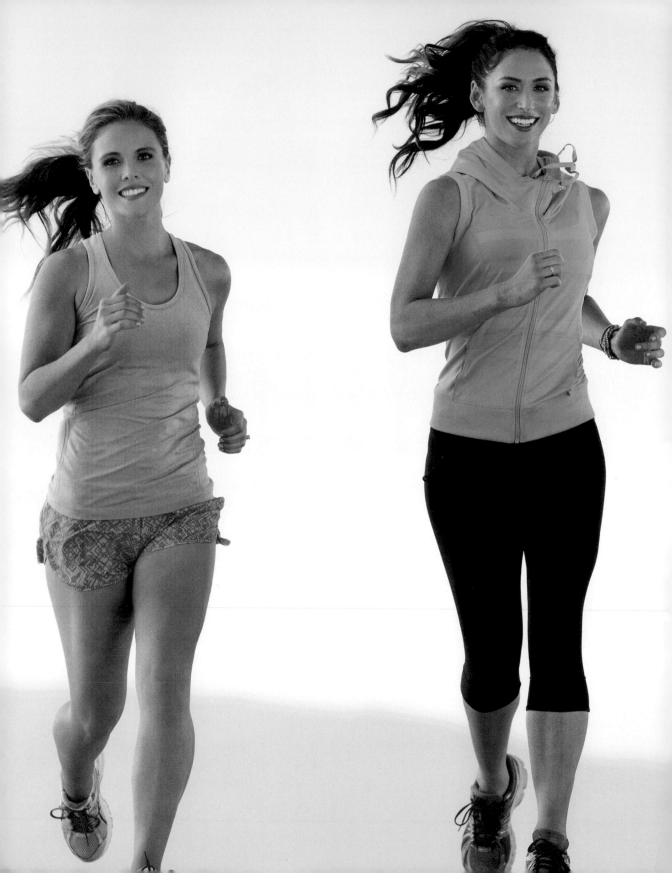

Part 5

The Workouts
Daily Fitness Challenges

Each week during your Fit, Fierce, and Fabulous challenge, you'll do two full-body strength-training routines, two HIIT (high-intensity interval training) routines, and two cardio routines. The routines change from week to week, to mix things up and get you the best result possible. As you progress through the program and your heart and muscles get stronger, your workouts will get increasingly more challenging. We'll kick up the reps, work multiple muscle groups at once (to save time and develop your "functional muscular fitness" for everyday life), and amp up your HIIT and cardio sessions to maximize your efforts and create a strong, knockout body!

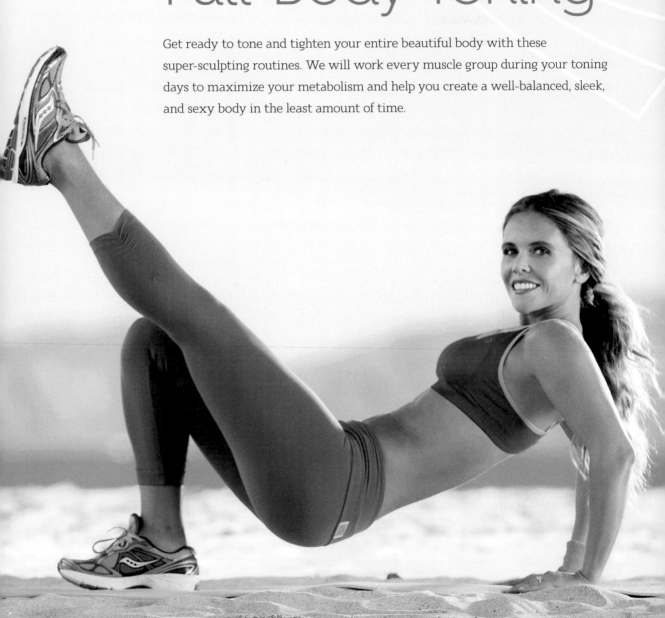

Full-Body Toning

Get ready to tone and tighten your entire beautiful body with these super-sculpting routines. We will work every muscle group during your toning days to maximize your metabolism and help you create a well-balanced, sleek, and sexy body in the least amount of time.

Sweet-and-Spicy Strength Training

In Week 1 of your training we're going to focus on large muscle groups like your legs, glutes, back, and abs. Strengthening these will lay a powerful foundation for all your future workouts. Plus, targeting these babies burns major calories and increases your metabolism all day long!

For each move, complete 3 sets of 12 to 14 reps. In between each set, take a 30-second break to catch your breath and take a sip of water. Complete all 3 sets of the same move before you move on to the next exercise.

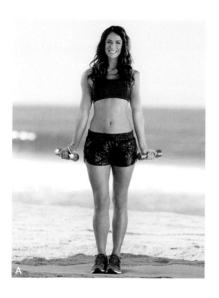

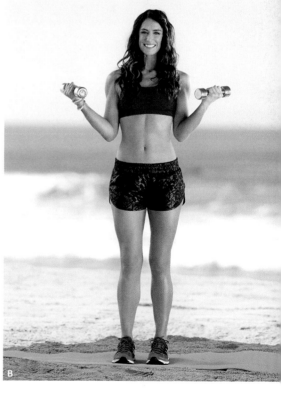

Bicep Curl

Standing tall with your abdominals engaged, hold a dumbbell in each hand by your sides, palms facing forward. Curl the weight up to your shoulders and return to the starting position, slow and controlled.

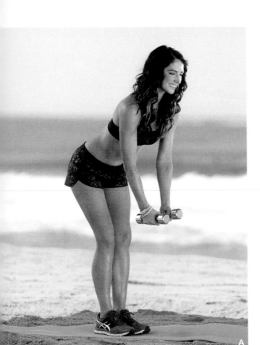

Tricep Kickback

With your feet hip distance apart, bend forward at the hips to about 45 degrees, keeping your abs engaged. Holding your dumbbells by your chest and your elbows tucked into your sides, extend your forearms back until they are parallel with the floor. Keeping your elbows stationary, with a slow and controlled motion, bring your dumbbells back to the starting position by your chest.

Bent-Over Rear Fly

With your feet hip distance apart, bend forward at the hips to about 45 degrees, keeping your abs engaged. Holding your dumbbells under your shoulders, slowly and with control, fly them back until they are parallel with the floor and in line with your midback. Be sure to keep your shoulders down away from your ears and your spine neutral.

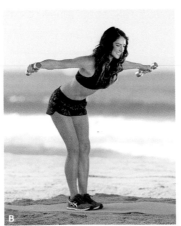

Upright Row

Begin in a standing position with your abs engaged. Hold your dumbbells straight down beneath your shoulders with your palms facing your body. Leading with your elbows, slowly raise your dumbbells until they reach your chest and your elbows are parallel to the floor. Make sure to keep your wrists neutral and your shoulders down and away from your ears.

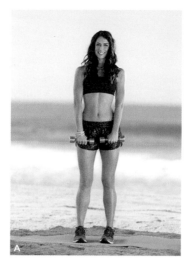

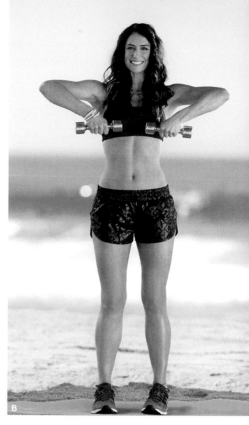

Squat

Stand with your feet shoulder width apart, abs engaged, and shoulders back. Bending at the hips, sit back with your booty as if you were going to sit in a chair. Make sure your knees stay in line with your ankles and do not extend over your toes. Keep your chest forward and your shoulders back. Then, driving all of your weight into your heels, stand back up into the starting position.

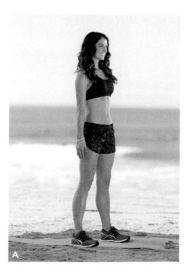

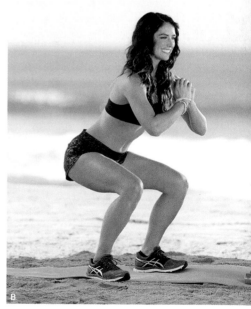

Curtsy Lunge

Begin with your feet shoulder width apart. Step back behind you into a curtsy with hands on your hips. Bend both knees until your front knee is at 90 degrees and does not drop in front of your toes. Drive your weight into your front heel to stand. Alternate sides.

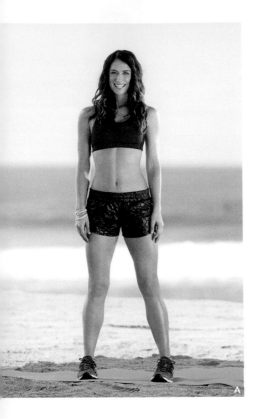

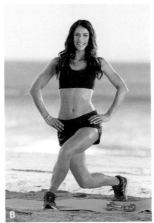

Back Lunge with a Twist

Stand with your feet shoulder width apart, holding one weight with both hands in front of your chest and engaging your abs. Step far back behind you with one leg, bending both knees to 90 degrees and dropping straight down while twisting your body toward the front leg. Drive all of your weight into your front heel to stand back up to the starting position. Alternate sides.

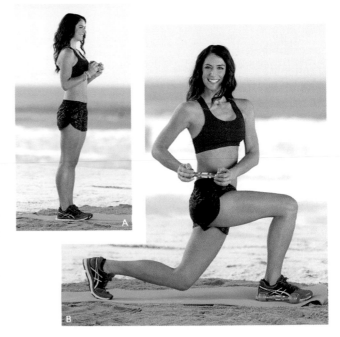

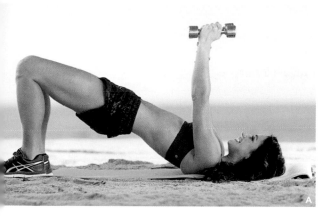

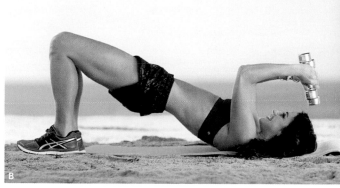

Booty Bridge with Tricep Extension

Lie on your back with your knees bent and feet flat on the floor, shoulder width apart, a dumbbell in each hand. Lift your booty up, making a straight line from your knees to your chest, then extend your arms straight out in front of your chest. Bend the elbows back at 90 degrees and extend back up, squeezing your triceps. Keep your hips high to the sky for all!

Booty Bridge Press

Lie on your back with your knees bent and feet flat on the floor, shoulder width apart, with your hips raised and a dumbbell in each hand. With your elbows wide and weights at chest level, press the weights to the sky. Return to the starting position, slowly and controlled, and repeat.

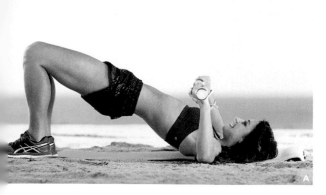

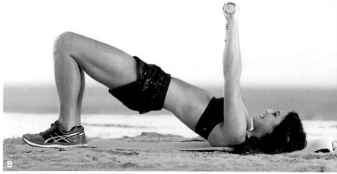

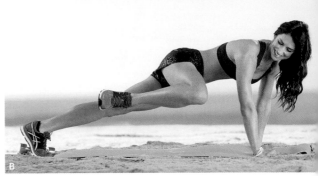

Tone It Up Tummy Toner

Align your body in a plank position, keeping your hips forward and core tight as you create a straight line from your shoulders through your hips to your ankles. Hold for a count of two here, then bring your right knee up toward your right elbow. Hold for a count of one and return your leg back into plank. Repeat as instructed, alternating sides.

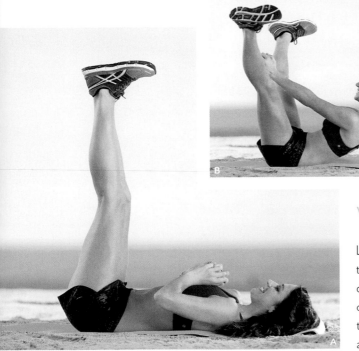

V Crunch

Lie on your back with legs straight and reaching to the sky, using both hands to hold one weight at your chest. Use your abs to sit up, abducting your legs out to the sides and pressing the weight between the legs. Return to the starting position and repeat as instructed.

WEEK 2

Magical Mermaid Moves

In Week 2, we're going to incorporate those multiple-muscle moves we were raving about. We're also going to increase your reps to 14 to 16, to turn up the heat and blast away fat to reveal sleek and sexy mermaid muscles!

Warrior 2 Lunge and Curl

With one dumbbell in each hand, stand with your feet wide and your left foot facing forward and bent at 90 degrees, back foot at 45 degrees. Glance to the left and lift your arms up at 90 degrees. Making sure the tailbone tucks toward the floor and your core is engaged with your hips facing forward, straighten your arms at the same time as you straighten your front leg. Return to the starting position and repeat reps on the other side.

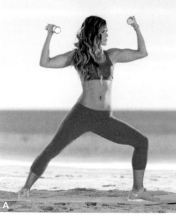

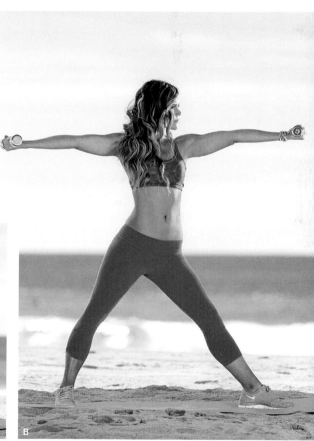

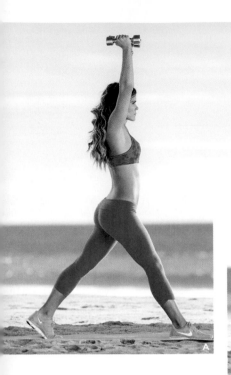

Sweeping Warrior 1

With one dumbbell in each hand, stand with your feet wide and your right foot facing forward, back foot at 45 degrees. Bend the front knee and hinge forward at the hips as you sweep your arms behind you. Slowly and with control, return to the starting position.

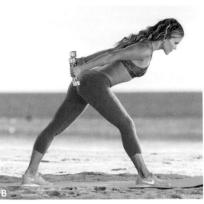

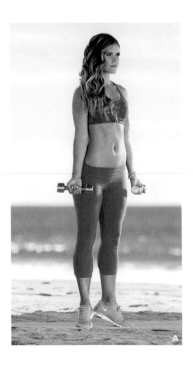

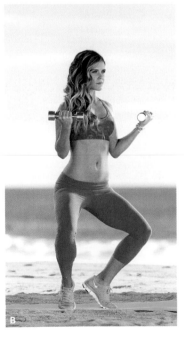

Plié and Curl

Begin on your tiptoes with your feet turned out 45 degrees and your heels kissing! Hold a dumbbell in each hand. Without moving your torso, bend at the knees while curling your dumbbells up to your chest. Return to the starting position.

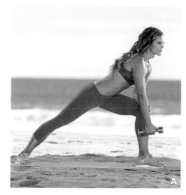

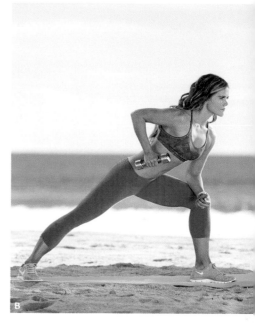

Bent-Over Row

Begin with your legs in a very wide stance and a dumbbell in your right hand. Bend over and rest your left elbow on your left thigh while you let your right arm hang to the floor. With your abs engaged, row your dumbbell up just below your chest. Complete reps on one side and then switch to the other.

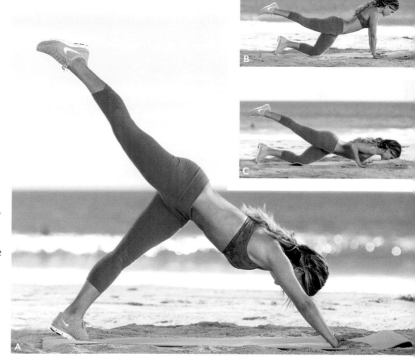

Downward-Dog Tricep Dip

Begin in a downward-dog position: body in an inverted V with your palms driving into the floor and hips to the sky. Lift one leg up to the sky while placing the other knee on the floor to perform a tricep pushup, keeping your lifted leg raised. Return to downward dog and alternate sides.

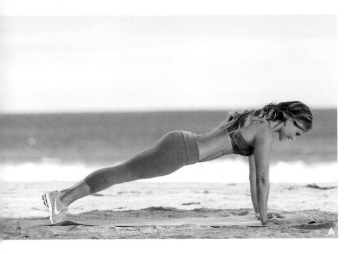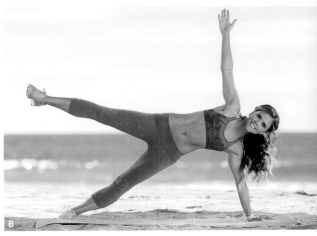

Starfish Plank

Begin in a high plank position with your hands in line with your shoulders. Rotate your entire body to balance in a side plank with your arm extended to the sky and your top leg lifted. If you need to modify this, you can keep both legs together in a straight line, or drop down to your bottom knee. Hold for one count and alternate sides.

Leg Abduction

Lying on your side, lift your top leg to the sky. Lower it back down slowly and controlled with abs engaged. Repeat reps on both sides.

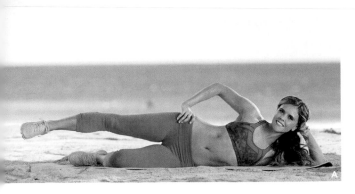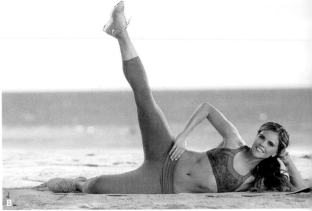

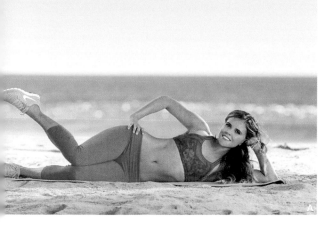
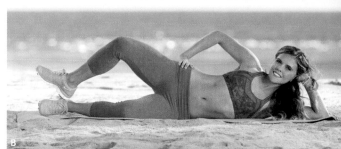

Clam

Lie on your side. Resting on your forearm or shoulder, bend both of your knees at 90 degrees and touch your knees together. Keeping your knees bent, rotate the hip and have your feet touch. This one burns, baby!

Clam Kick

Lie on your side. Resting on your forearm or shoulder, bend both of your knees at 90 degrees. Touch your knees together and then kick your top leg to the sky. Return to the starting position with your knees touching. Complete your reps and repeat on the other side.

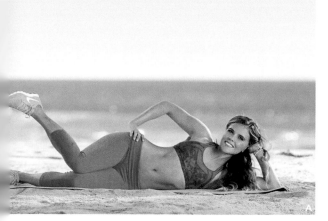
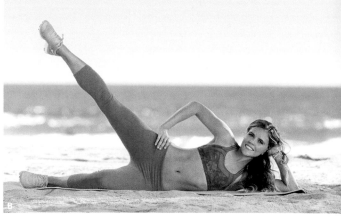

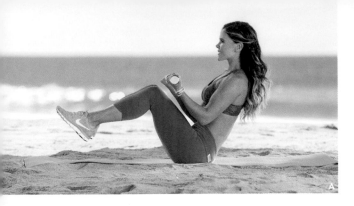

V-Sit Curl

Sit on the ground with your dumbbells close to your chest and your knees bent directly under the dumbbells. Extend your legs out at the same time you extend your dumbbells, while keeping your abs engaged. Return to the starting position by curling your dumbbells to your chest and bringing your legs in.

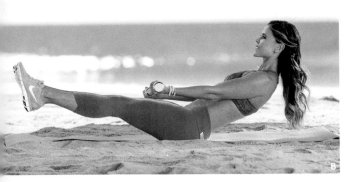

Plank Crunch with Glute Kickback

Begin in a high plank position with your spine neutral, abs engaged, and hands in line with your shoulders. Slowly and with control, lift your right leg while squeezing your glutes. Bring your right knee to your nose while squeezing your abs. Complete reps on one side and then switch sides.

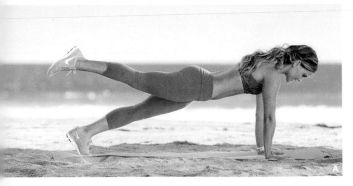
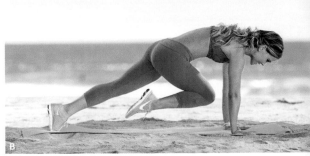

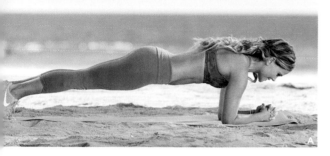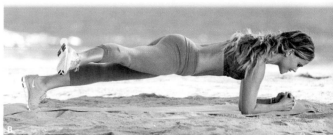

Forearm-Plank Toe Touch

Begin in a forearm plank position. Keeping your spine neutral and your abs engaged, lift and abduct one leg at a time out to the side. Alternate sides. Remember to breathe!

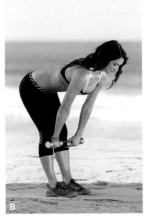

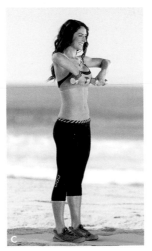

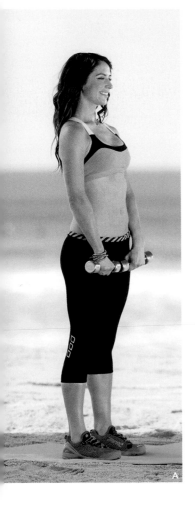

Bombshell Bonanza

In Week 3, our focus is on building strength, so pick up a heavier set of weights. If you've been using 5-pound dumbbells, increase to 8 pounds, 10 pounds, or even 12 pounds—whatever feels good for you and your level. Do 16 to 20 reps of each move in the circuit and repeat the circuit 3 times total. Take a 60-second break in between each circuit to catch your breath and take a sip of water.

Deadlift to Upright Row

Stand tall with dumbbells in your hands and palms facing toward your body and lightly resting on the front of your hips. With a flat back, slowly hinge forward at the hips as you allow the weights to gently slide down the front of your quads toward your shins until you feel a stretch in the backs of your legs. Maintaining a flat back, slowly rise from this position using the backs of your legs to pull your upper body upright and finish by pressing forward through your hips, with your weights back at the front of your hips.

From the returned upright position, engage your core and lower your shoulders back and down as you pull your elbows up to eye level at your sides. Keep the weight below your elbows and almost tucked into your armpits. Hold for one count and slowly lower down to the starting position. Repeat both movements as instructed.

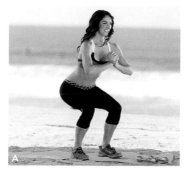

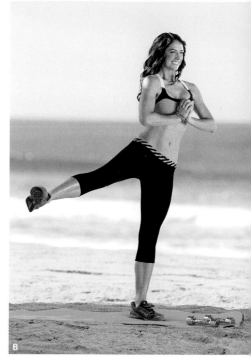

Squat to Hip Abduction

Stand tall with your feet shoulder width apart. With a flat back and hands clasped in front of your chest, sit back with your weight in your heels as you let your booty drop toward the floor. Make sure to keep your knees directly in line with your toes as you bring your quads as close to parallel with the floor as possible. Squeeze your abs as you press down through your heels to stand back up, favoring your left leg as your legs straighten out. Kick your right leg out and up to your side. Lower your leg and repeat for the other side as instructed.

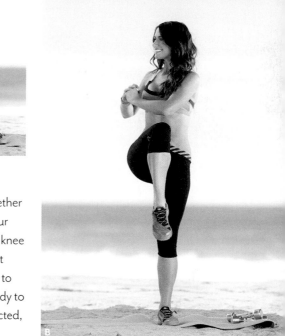

Side Lunge and Knee-Up Twist

Stand tall with your feet together, core tight, and hands clasped together in front of your chest. Step your left foot out to the side, bending your right knee and lunging down and keeping your booty back and your knee in line with your toes. Lower as far as you can, returning to an upright position by pressing down into your right heel. Before you step back to center, tuck your right knee up and forward and twist your upper body to the right to bring your left elbow to your right knee. Repeat as instructed, alternating sides.

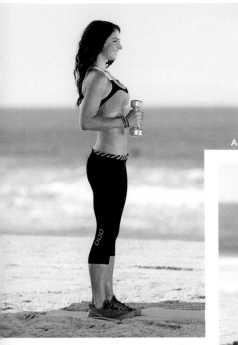

Forward Lunge and Tricep Kickback

Stand tall with your feet together and your arms bent at 90 degrees, holding your weights in front of you. Step forward with your right leg into a forward lunge, keeping your right knee in line with your toes.

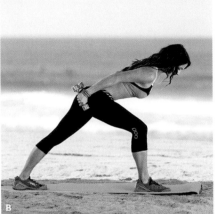

Bend slightly forward at the hips to allow your elbows to pull straight back to parallel with the ground, then kick your weights back behind you, straightening at the elbows. Return the weights to their forward position and press into your right heel to stand back up. Repeat as instructed, alternating sides.

The Heat Wave

Lie on your back with your knees bent to 90 degrees, feet under your knees. Press up through your heels and forward through your hips to create a straight line from your knees through your hips to your shoulders. Twist your hips side to side by pressing down through your right heel and lifting your hips to your right, then alternating to your left. Repeat as instructed.

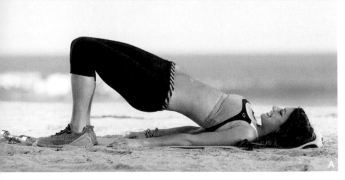

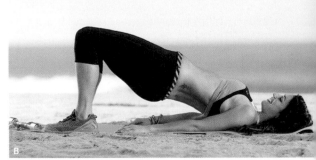

Boat-Pose Curl and Press

Sit on your mat in boat pose and hold your weights down by your hips with your palms facing the sky. Curl the weights up to your shoulders, then rotate your shoulders out so that your weights are out to your sides and directly above your elbows. Press up through the heels of your palms to straighten your arms overhead. Slowly lower the weights back down to eye level, then rotate your shoulders in as you bring your elbows to your sides. Lower the weight down to your hips again.

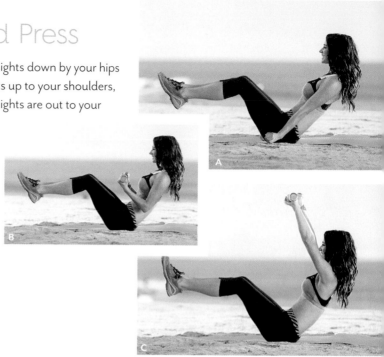

Bicycle Twist

Sit on your mat in boat pose holding one dumbbell in front of your chest. With a flat back, twist your upper body to the left as you tuck your left leg up to bring your left knee to meet your right elbow. Kick your left leg back out and twist to your right as your tuck your right knee up to meet your left elbow. Repeat as instructed.

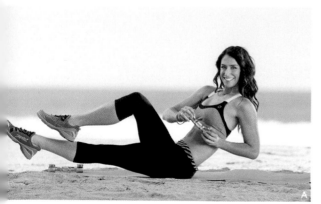

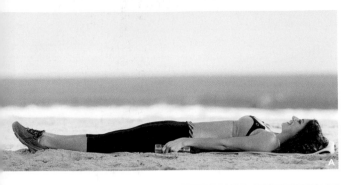

Single-Leg Straight-Legged V Sit with Alternating Bicep Curl

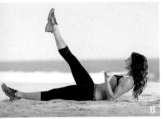
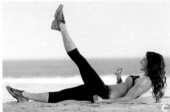

Lie on your back with weights in your hands. With your palms facing the sky, perform a crunch as you pull your right leg straight up to the sky, simultaneously doing a bicep curl with your left arm. Hold for one count and slowly lower back down to the mat. Repeat for the opposite side by performing a crunch as you pull your left leg straight up to the sky and do a bicep curl with your right arm. Again lower back down to your mat and repeat as instructed.

Superwoman and Row

Lie on your stomach with arms stretched out overhead, feet shoulder width apart. Squeeze your lower back and booty as you lift your knees and chest off the mat, reaching to the horizon with your hands and feet. Slowly row your elbows back parallel with the ground, keeping your hands off the mat, until your elbows are tucked back to your side. Hold for one count and then stretch your arms back overhead before lowering your knees and chest to the mat again. Repeat as instructed.

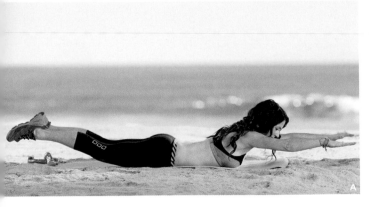
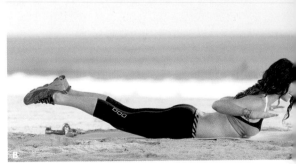

Rock It Like You Mean It

It's Week 4: time to really push through and build those long, lean muscles with high reps! These moves target every single muscle fiber, big and small. Stick with the same amount of weight you used in Week 3. Complete 1 set of 25 reps for each move and then 2 more sets of 18 to 20 reps each. This week burns, but the results are so worth it! Take a 60-second break in between sets.

Squat and Curl

Stand tall with weights in your hands, arms resting at your sides. With a flat back, sit back with your weight in your heels as you let your booty drop toward the floor. Make sure to keep your knees directly in line with your toes as you bring your quads as close to parallel with the floor as possible, keeping the weights at your sides with straight arms. Squeeze your abs as you press down through your heels to stand back up and press forward through your hips.

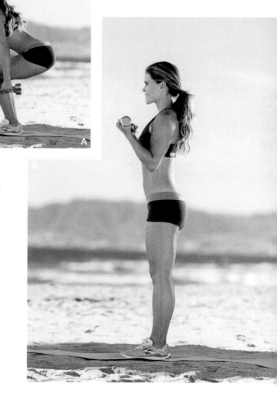

Once standing upright, curl the weights up to your shoulders. Lower the weights down to your hips again. Repeat as instructed.

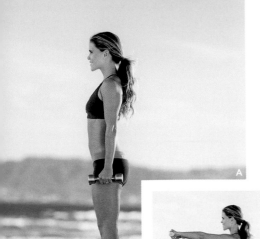

Reverse Lunge and Front Raise

Stand tall with your feet together, holding your weights down in front of you, palms facing in. Step backward with your right leg into a reverse lunge, keeping your left knee in line with your left toes and your right knee directly under your hips. Lower your right knee straight down to the ground as you raise your weights straight forward and up with straight arms, bringing them out in front of you at eye level. Press down through your front heel to stand back up as you slowly lower your weights back down to your sides. Repeat as instructed.

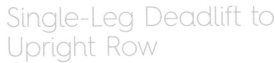

Single-Leg Deadlift to Upright Row

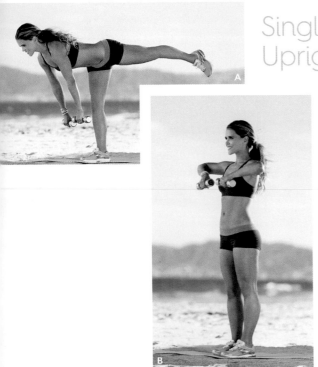

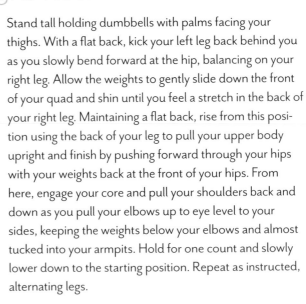

Stand tall holding dumbbells with palms facing your thighs. With a flat back, kick your left leg back behind you as you slowly bend forward at the hip, balancing on your right leg. Allow the weights to gently slide down the front of your quad and shin until you feel a stretch in the back of your right leg. Maintaining a flat back, rise from this position using the back of your leg to pull your upper body upright and finish by pushing forward through your hips with your weights back at the front of your hips. From here, engage your core and pull your shoulders back and down as you pull your elbows up to eye level to your sides, keeping the weights below your elbows and almost tucked into your armpits. Hold for one count and slowly lower down to the starting position. Repeat as instructed, alternating legs.

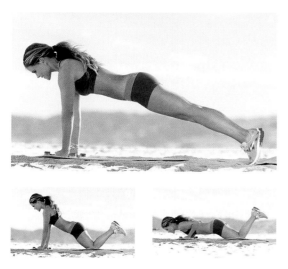

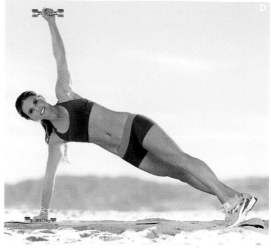

Tricep Pushup, Row, and Twist

Drop down to your mat into a pushup position with weights in hand, holding your body in a plank, creating a straight line from your shoulders through your hips to your feet (or knees). Perform a tricep pushup by lowering yourself down with your arms, keeping your shoulders down and elbows tucked into your waist-line. Once your hips are almost touching your mat, press the heel of your palms into the mat to rise again, and balancing on your feet and right hand, row your left arm back as you rotate your hips to your left, stacking your feet and then pressing your left arm to the sky above your body, creating a letter T. Hold for one count and slowly lower back down to the mat. Repeat as instructed, alternating sides.

Crab Up

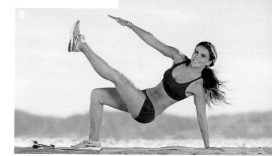

Sit on your mat with your knees bent at 90 degrees and your feet on the ground. Place your hands on the mat beneath your elbows, pressing forward through your hips to lift them up, pressing down into the mat with your hands and the heel of your right foot. As your hips reach to the sky, kick your left leg out and up and crunch it up as you reach your right arm out to touch your left toes, balancing on your right leg and left arm. Hold for a count of one and slowly lower back down to the mat. Repeat as instructed, alternating sides.

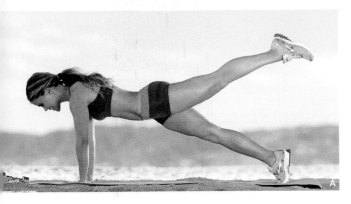
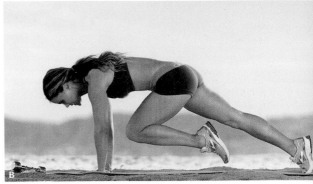

Plank to Knee Tuck

Align your body in a plank position, keeping your hips forward and core tight as you create a straight line from your shoulders through your hips to your ankles. Raise your left leg up, keeping the core and glutes engaged. Hold for a count of two here, then tuck your left knee up underneath you as you round your back slightly. Hold for a count of one and return your leg back into plank. Repeat as instructed, alternating sides.

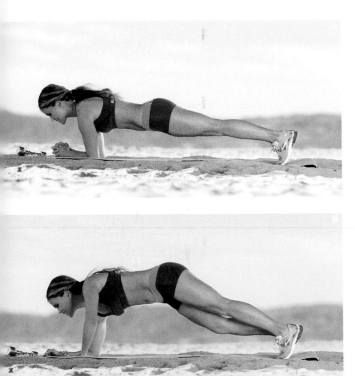

Alternating Plank

Align your body in a plank position, keeping your hips forward and core tight as you create a straight line from your shoulders through your hips to your ankles. Hold tight here as you breathe. Place your weight on your left hand as you rotate gently onto your right forearm, followed by your left forearm. Hold for a count of two and press back to your hands, keeping your hips from rotating as much as possible. Repeat as instructed, alternating sides.

High-Intensity Interval Training (HIIT)

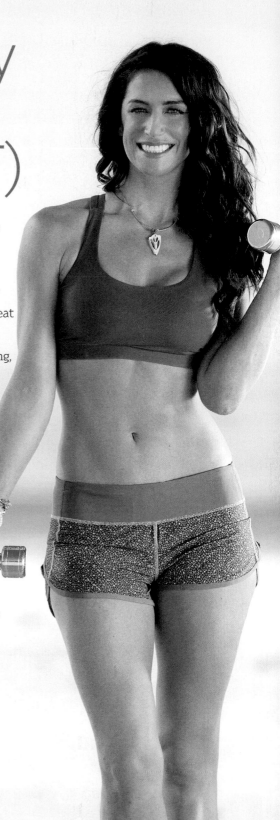

For firing up metabolism and revving energy, nothing beats high-intensity interval training!

Why is HIIT so great? It's in the science. This type of training combines periods of high intensity mixed with low intensity and causes your body to work hard after your sweat session to build up its oxygen stores. This means more bang for your buck! Who doesn't want to burn calories all day long, even when not working out? This process is called excess post-exercise oxygen consumption, or EPOC, and it's the reason why you're still sweating even after you cool down and shower. Regular HIIT workouts turn your body into a lean, fat-burning machine!

Here's an important tip: Work as hard as you possibly can during your high-intensity cardio intervals. The fabulous burning sensation you feel is a signal that you've hit your fat-blasting anaerobic zone. Listen to your body and take a water break whenever you need it.

Note: Always warm up and cool down for at least 5 minutes before and after each HIIT session.

Burn, Baby, Burn

In Week 1, we are building our base for HIIT. This is your 20-minute beginner HIIT routine. Repeat this circuit 2 times, resting for 30 to 60 seconds in between circuits.

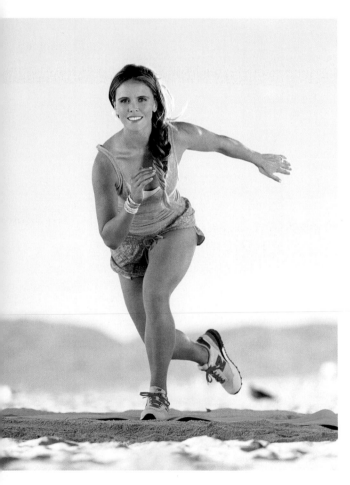

Skater

Stand on your mat with legs together and arms by your sides. Begin by balancing on your left leg and bending it slightly. Tuck your right leg behind you and bring your right arm up in front of you with your elbow bent at 90 degrees like you are in the middle of a run or skate. Jump from your left leg to your right leg and adjust your body's position accordingly to maintain balance as you "skate" side to side. Repeat as instructed for 45 seconds.

One-Legged Shoulder Abduction

Stand tall on your left leg with your right leg behind you, toe on the ground if needed for balance. Grasp one weight in each hand and hold them at your hips, palms facing forward. Squeeze your abs tight and lift the weights up to 45-degree angles at 10 o'clock and 2 o'clock, creating a circle from your hips to overhead. Hold for a count of one and slowly lower down to the starting position. Repeat as instructed, alternating legs, for 30 seconds. Rest for 15 seconds.

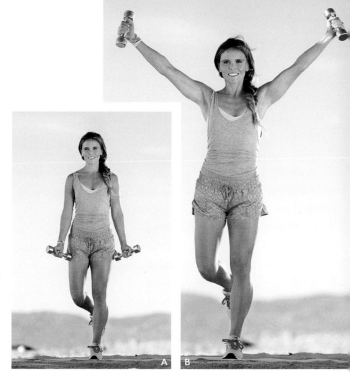

Standing Straight-Leg Bicycle Crunch

Stand tall with your feet shoulder width apart, with your arms stretched out by your sides. Begin by lifting your right leg up in front of you, keeping your knee straight. Pull your leg up to hip level as you reach your left arm across your body to touch your right foot. Slowly lower back down to the starting position. Repeat as instructed, alternating sides, for 45 seconds.

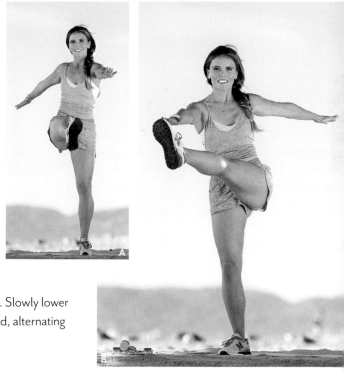

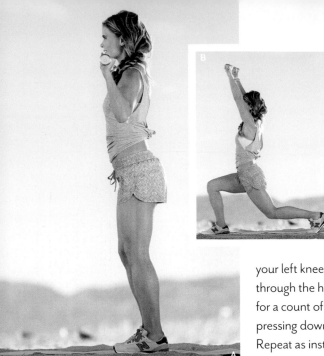

Forward Lunge and Shoulder Press

Stand tall with your feet together. Holding your weights in your hands, lift your arms up by your sides, elbows bent to 90 degrees, wrists directly over your elbows. Step forward with your right leg into a lunge, keeping your right knee in line with your toes and your left knee directly under your hips. Lower your left knee straight down to the ground as you press your weights up through the heels of your palms to straighten your arms overhead. Hold for a count of one and slowly lower back down to the starting position, pressing down into the heel of your forward leg to stand back up. Repeat as instructed, alternating sides, for a total of 30 seconds.

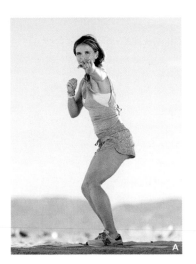
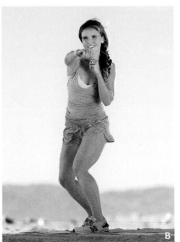
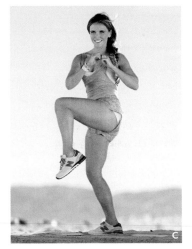

Tone It Up Punch and Crunch

Standing in the middle of your mat, place one foot out in front of the other in an athletic stance and bring your hands up in front of your face. Begin by punching your left hand forward, rotating your body as you pull your left hand back in to protect your face, and punch your right arm forward. Rotate back, pivoting on your back leg as you punch your left hand forward, once again pulling your hands back in front of your face and your front knee up to your torso, working the abs. Repeat for 30 seconds on each side for a total of 60 seconds.

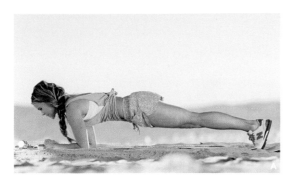 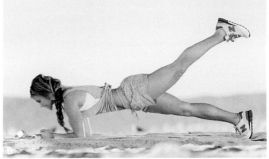

Forearm Plank with Alternating Kickback

Align your body in a forearm plank position, keeping your hips forward and core tight as you create a straight line from your shoulders through your hips to your ankles. Hold tight here as you breathe. Place your weight on your right foot as you kick your left leg straight back and up, squeezing your booty. Try to keep your hips from rotating as much as possible. Repeat as instructed, alternating sides, for 30 seconds.

Single-Leg Booty Bridge with Chest Press

Lie down on your back with weights in your hands. Bend your left knee to 90 degrees, with your foot directly underneath your knee. Kick your right leg straight up into the air. Bend your elbows to 90 degrees, with your elbows on the mat and your weights in the air directly above your elbows. From here, press down into the mat to lift your booty into the air. Press forward through your hips as you press forward into the palms of your hands to perform a chest press, bringing your elbows together in front of you, keeping the weight directly above your elbows at all times. Hold for a count of one, then slowly lower your booty back down to your mat. Repeat as instructed for 30 seconds on each side, for a total of 60 seconds.

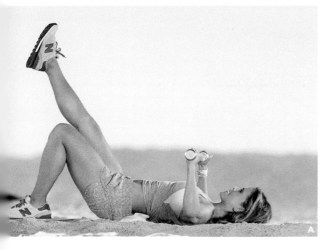 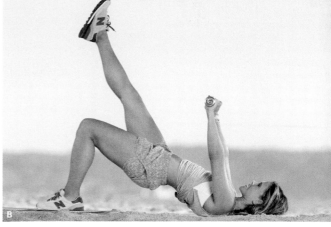

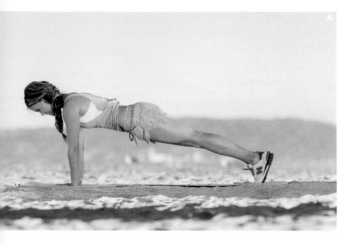

Alternating Jump Tuck—45 seconds

Align your body in a plank position. Keeping your hands firmly planted, hop your feet up under your hips by tucking your knees up to your chest. Kick your feet back out to your right side and hold that side plank for a count of one. Hop your feet back up under your hips and kick them back out to your left side. Hold for a count of one, hop them back up, and kick straight back again. Repeat all three directions as instructed for 45 seconds. Rest for 15 seconds.

NOTE: You'll do this move twice in this routine, 45 seconds the first time and 60 seconds the second time.

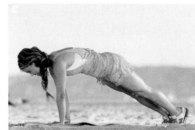

Rainbow

Come down onto your mat on your right hand and right hip. Stack your feet, place your hip on the mat, and keep your right arm straight. With your left arm up above your head, pull your hips up off the mat, extending by lifting your hips as high as you can and allowing your arm to hang over your head. Hold for a count of one and slowly lower your hips back down to your mat. Repeat for 30 seconds on each side for a total of 60 seconds.

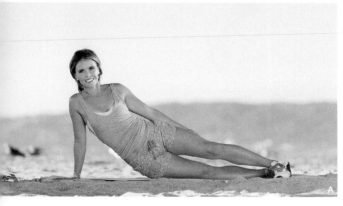

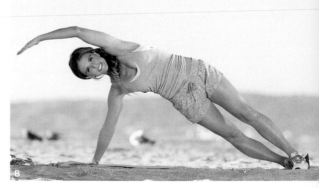

Tricep Pushup

Align your body in a plank position, keeping your hips forward and core tight as you create a straight line from your shoulders through your hips to your ankles. Perform a tricep pushup by lowering yourself down with your arms, keeping your shoulders down and elbows tucked into your waistline. Once your hips are almost touching your mat, press the heel of your palms into the mat and fully extend your elbows to return to a plank position. Repeat as instructed for 30 seconds.

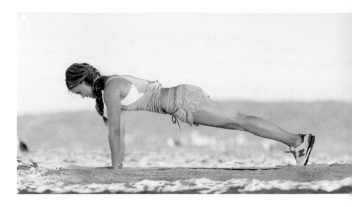

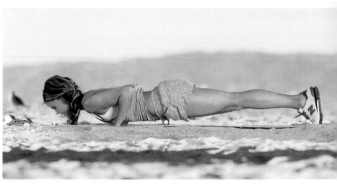

Alternating Jump Tuck— 60 seconds

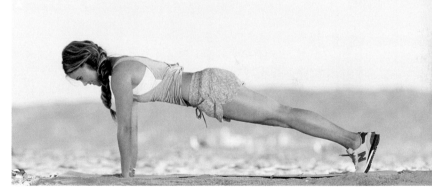

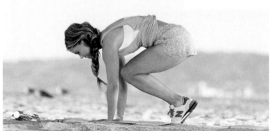

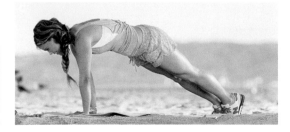

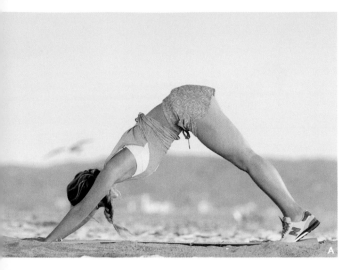

Downward-Upward Dog

Start this move in downward-facing dog. Hands are shoulder width apart, palms are flat, and fingers are spread. Feet are hip width apart with heels aiming toward the ground. Your spine is long. Leave a slight bend in the knees to protect the lower back. Slowly transition into upward-facing dog.

Hands are shoulder width apart, arms are straight, thighs are lifted off the floor, and you rest on the tops of your feet. Lift your chest up and bring your shoulders down and back. Finish by lifting your booty back up into downward-facing dog, using your abs. Repeat this move for a total of 60 seconds.

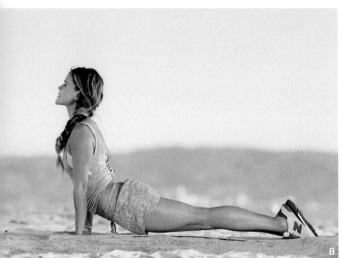

WEEK 2

Shred and Shine

In Week 2, we are increasing our cardio spurts and toning moves to build endurance. Try doing this routine straight, breaking only between the two circuits. The toning moves worked in here will bring your heart rate down and serve as active rest.

Workout time: 26 minutes
Perform each move below for 60 seconds!

Switch-Back Jump Squat

Stand tall with your feet shoulder width apart. With a flat back, sit back with your weight in your heels as you let your booty drop toward the floor. Make sure to keep your knees directly in line with your toes as you bring your quads as close to parallel with the floor as possible. Squeeze your abs as you press down through your heels and drive down into the ground to jump up while turning 180 degrees in the air and landing with soft knees facing the opposite direction. Repeat by continuing to switch sides.

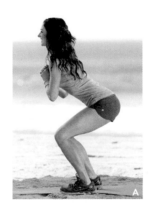

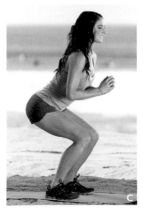

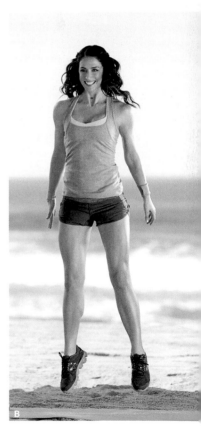

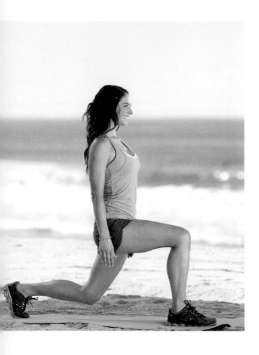

Lunge

Stand tall with your feet together and your arms at your sides. Step forward with your right leg into a forward lunge, keeping your right knee in line with your toes and your left knee directly under your hips. Lower your left knee straight down to the ground as you bend slightly forward at the hips. Hold for a count of one, then press into your right heel to stand back up. Repeat as instructed, alternating sides.

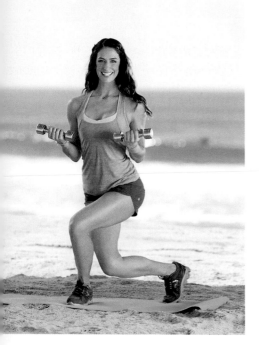

Curtsy Lunge and Curl

Stand tall with your feet together, holding dumbbells at your sides. Step back with your right leg, tucking your right knee behind your left leg into a curtsy lunge, keeping your left knee in line with your left toes and your right knee directly under your right hip. Lower your right knee straight down to the ground. Perform a curl with your dumbbells at the same time. Hold for a count of one, then press into your left heel to stand back up. Repeat as instructed, alternating sides.

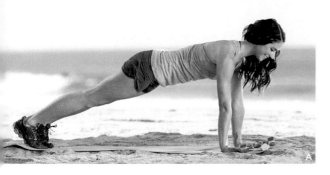

Plank Jack

Come down onto your mat in a plank position, with your hands stretched out under your shoulders. Support your weight with your legs together and straight back behind you and your hips forward. Squeeze your abs. Jump your feet out to wider than shoulder width apart and then jump them back in together. Repeat as instructed.

Plank and Row

Drop down to your mat into a pushup position with a weight in your right hand, holding yourself up with your left arm stretched out under your shoulder, creating a straight line from your shoulders through your hips to your feet (or knees). Pull your right elbow back and into your side, rowing the weight while keeping your hips square to your mat. Hold for a count of one and slowly lower the weight back down to the mat. Repeat as instructed, alternating sides.

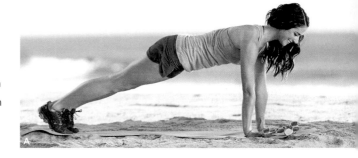

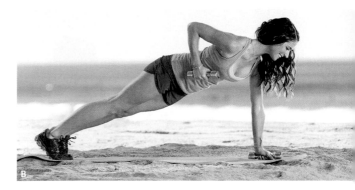

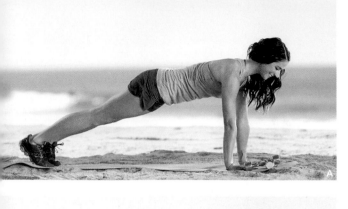

Tone It Up
Tummy Toner

Align your body in a plank position, keeping your hips forward and core tight as you create a straight line from your shoulders through your hips to your ankles. Hold for a count of two here, then bring your right knee up toward your right elbow. Hold for a count of one and return your leg back into plank. Repeat as instructed, alternating sides.

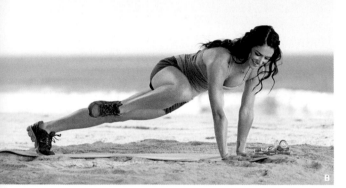

Mountain Climber

Align your body in a plank position, keeping your hips forward and core tight as you create a straight line from your shoulders through your hips to your ankles. Tuck your right knee up toward your chest, and in one swift movement, kick your right leg back as you tuck your left leg up to your chest, keeping your booty low. Repeat as instructed, alternating sides.

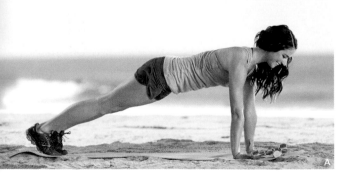

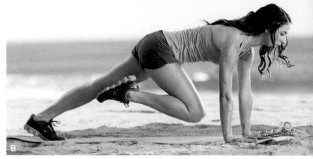

Tricep Pushup

Align your body in a plank position, keeping your hips forward, core tight, and knees touching the ground. Perform a tricep pushup by lowering yourself down with your arms, keeping your shoulders down and elbows tucked into your waistline. Once your hips are almost touching your mat, press the heel of your palms into the mat to rise again. Repeat as instructed.

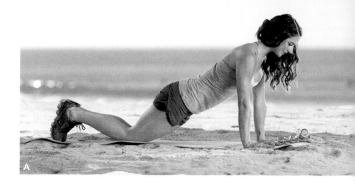

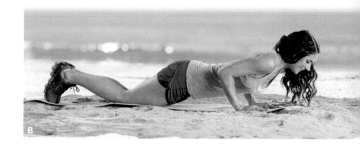

Flip Out

From downward-facing dog, lift your right leg up and stack your right hip on top of your left. Slowly continue rotating so that your right toes find the floor. When stable, reach your right hand overhead and lift your chest. Flip back to downward-facing dog when finished. Repeat on the other side.

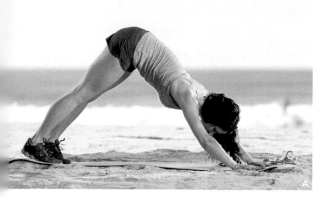

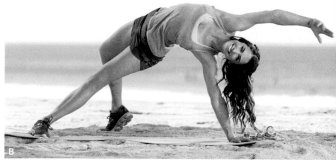

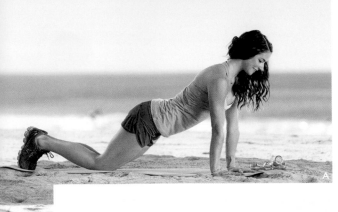

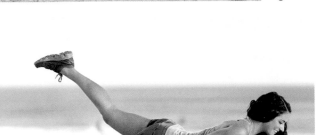

Tricep Pushup and Kickback

Align your body in a plank position, keeping your hips forward, core tight, and knees touching the ground. Perform a tricep pushup by lowering yourself down with your arms, keeping your shoulders down and elbows tucked into your waistline. Once your hips are almost touching your mat, press the heel of your palms into the mat to rise again and kick your left leg back behind you, squeezing your booty. Hold for a count of one and place your foot back on the mat. Repeat as instructed, alternating legs.

Bicycle Crunch

Lie on your mat with your knees bent to 90 degrees, feet directly under your knees. Place your hands behind your neck with your elbows out to your sides. Crunch your shoulders up and twist your upper body to the left as you tuck your left leg up to bring your left knee to meet your right elbow. Kick your left leg back out and twist to your right as you tuck your right knee up to meet your left elbow. Repeat as instructed.

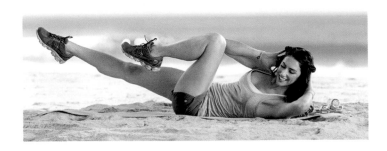

Burpee

Stand tall at the front of your mat. Reach down to the floor and place your hands by the outsides of your feet. Jump your feet backward to the back of your mat so that you land in a plank position. Hold for a count of one and jump your knees back up so that you land at the front of your mat. From here, adjust yourself into a squat position and drive down through your heels to jump up, reaching as high as possible. Land with soft knees and repeat as instructed.

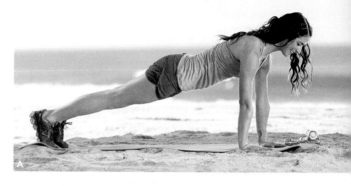

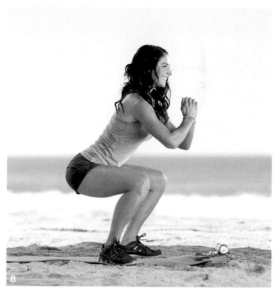

3

Rev Up and Rock Out

This week we are revving up! Time to increase your weights during your HIIT, same as in your full-body strength-training workouts. If you were using 5 pounds, switch to 8 pounds, or 8 pounds to 10 pounds, and so on. Do this circuit twice, resting for 60 seconds between circuits. These 30 minutes are heart pumping—get ready to sweat!

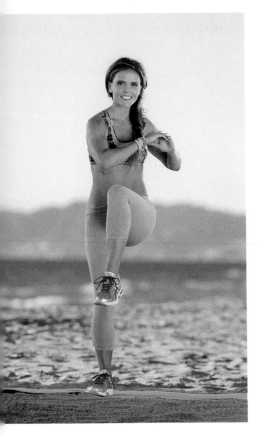

Alternating Jump Crunch

Stand on your mat with your feet shoulder width apart and clasp your hands together in front of your chest. Begin by balancing on your right leg and tucking your left knee up as you twist your body left to bring your right elbow to meet your left knee. Repeat as instructed, alternating sides., for 60 seconds.

Standing Bicep Curl

Stand on your left foot with your right leg lifted at a 90-degree angle, hands by your sides and holding weights with palms facing forward. Squeeze your biceps as you curl the weights out to your sides and up, keeping your elbows tucked into your sides. Slowly lower the weights down to your sides. Repeat as instructed, for 60 seconds.

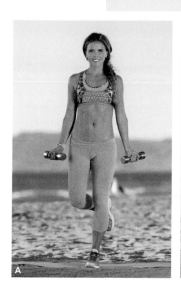
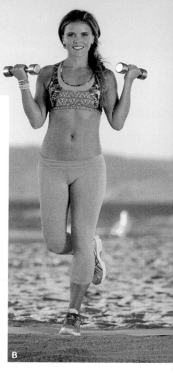

Standing Tricep Kickback

Stand tall with your feet together and bend slightly forward at the hips. Allow your elbows to pull straight back to parallel with the ground, then kick your weights back behind you, straightening the elbows. Slowly return the weights to their original position. Repeat as instructed, for 60 seconds.

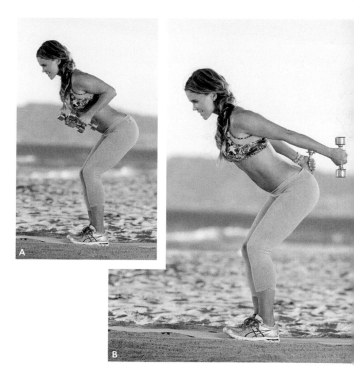

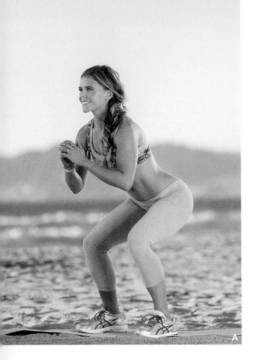
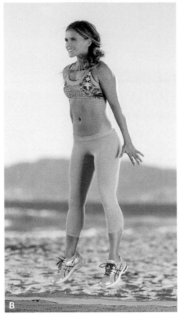

Jump Squat

Stand tall with your feet shoulder width apart. With a flat back, sit back with your weight in your heels as you let your booty drop toward the floor. Make sure to keep your knees directly in line with your toes as you bring your quads as close to parallel with the floor as possible. Squeeze your abs as you press down through your heels and drive into the ground to jump up, landing with soft knees. Repeat as instructed, for 60 seconds.

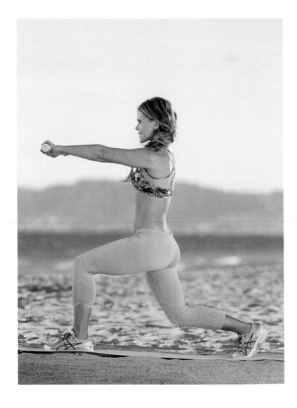

Reverse Lunge with Front Raise

Stand tall with your feet together, holding your weights down in front of you, palms facing inward. Step backward with your right leg into a reverse lunge, keeping your left knee in line with your toes and your right knee directly under your hips. Lower your right knee straight down to the ground as you raise your weights forward and up with straight arms, bringing them in front of you to shoulder level. Press down through your front heel to stand back up as you slowly lower your weights back down in front of you. Repeat as instructed, alternating sides, for 60 seconds.

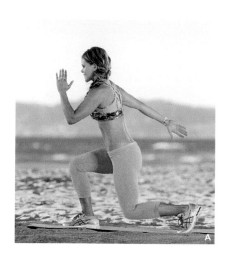
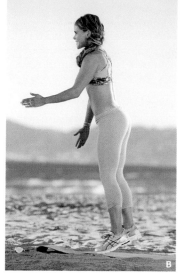
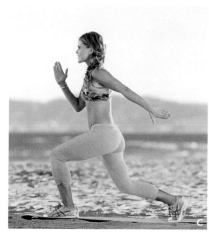

Plyo Lunge

Stand on your mat and step your right foot out to lunge down, keeping your booty back and your right knee in line with your right toes. Lunge down as far as you can and explode back up by pressing down into your right heel and launching yourself into the air. While in the air, switch your legs so that you land with your left leg forward and right leg back. Repeat as instructed, alternating sides, for 60 seconds.

Bent-Over Row and Booty Kickback

Stand on your mat with weights held by your sides and palms facing inward. Balance on your right foot as you bring your left leg back behind you, hinging slightly forward at the hips and allowing your arms to hang freely under your shoulders with your weights in hand. Pull your elbows up to your sides, performing a row as you kick your left leg upward behind you to squeeze your booty. Slowly lower your arms and leg back to the starting position. Complete reps on one side, for 45 seconds, and then switch sides, for another 45 seconds.

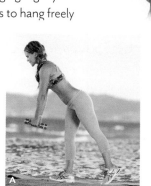
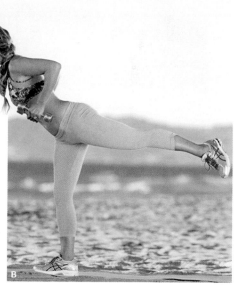

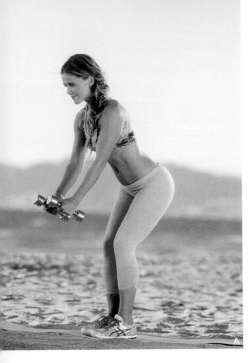

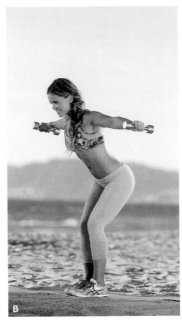

Reverse Fly

Stand with your feet together and bend slightly at the hips. Hold your weights out in front of you, allowing them to hang freely under your shoulders. Squeeze your abs as you pull your shoulder blades together and pull the weights back and up, opening your chest. Hold for a count of one with your arms out to your sides, then slowly lower the weights back down. Repeat as instructed, for 60 seconds.

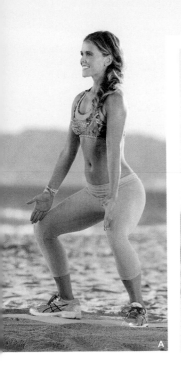

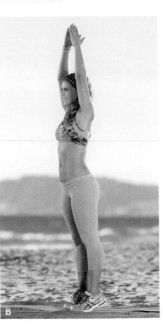

Plié Jumping Jack

Stand tall with your feet wider than shoulder width apart, toes pointed out to the sides, wrists resting on the front of your knees. With a flat back, sit back with your weight in your heels as you let your booty drop toward the floor, allowing your knees to track outward to perform a plié squat. Make sure to keep your knees directly in line with your toes as you bring your quads as close to parallel with the floor as possible. From this lowered position, drive into your heels to jump into the air, landing with your feet together and your arms overhead. Jump back into the air, this time landing back into the plié squat with your arms again resting in front of your knees. Repeat as instructed, for 90 seconds.

Row and Twist

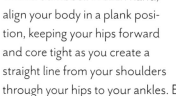

With a dumbbell in each hand, align your body in a plank position, keeping your hips forward and core tight as you create a straight line from your shoulders through your hips to your ankles. Balancing on your feet and right hand, row your left arm back as you rotate your hips to your left, stacking your feet and then pressing your left arm to the sky above your body, creating a letter T. Hold for a count of one and slowly lower back down to the mat in plank position. (Bonus: Lift your top leg and hold for one count.) Repeat as instructed, alternating sides, for 60 seconds.

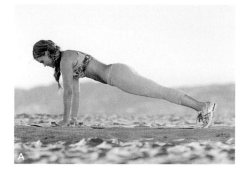
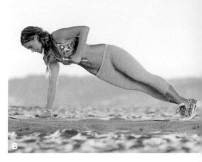

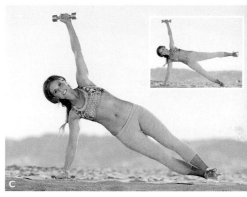

Alternating Plank

Align your body in a plank position, keeping your hips forward and core tight as you create a straight line from your shoulders through your hips to your ankles. Hold tight here as you breathe. Place your weight on your right hand as you rotate gently onto your left forearm, followed by your right forearm. Hold for a count of two and return back to your hands, keeping your hips from rotating as much as possible as you move from forearm plank to regular plank on your hands. Repeat as instructed, for 60 seconds.

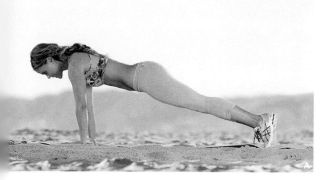
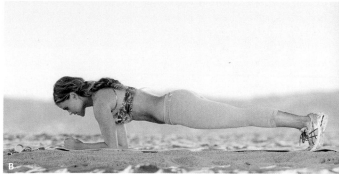

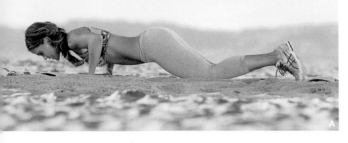

Plyo Pushup

Align your body in a plank position, keeping your hips forward and core tight as you create a straight line from your shoulders through your hips to your ankles. Perform a plyo pushup by lowering yourself down with your arms, keeping your shoulders down and elbows out. Once your hips are almost touching your mat, press into the heel of your palms and drive up. Clap at top! Repeat as instructed, for 90 seconds.

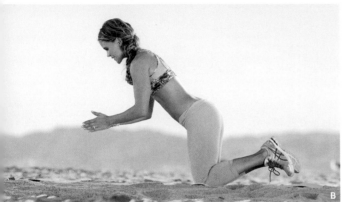

Mountain Climber

Align your body in a plank position, keeping your hips forward and core tight as you create a straight line from your shoulders through your hips to your ankles. Tuck your right knee up toward your chest and in one swift movement, kick your right leg back as you tuck your left leg up to your chest, keeping your booty low. Repeat as instructed, alternating sides, for 90 seconds.

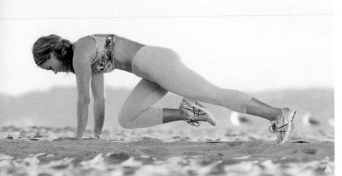

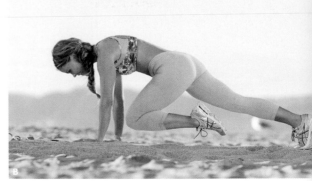

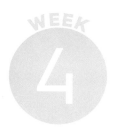

HIIT the High Note

This week we are taking it to the next level. Week 4 is intense, but you're primed and ready! We promise you're going to see some major results and definition. Your cardio bursts will be longer, but you will have plenty of time to rest, recover, and grab some water after your active toning moves.

Repeat each of the four circuits below twice and rest for 60 seconds before moving on to the next circuit. Each circuit has two toning moves and one cardio move.

Workout time: 37 intense minutes

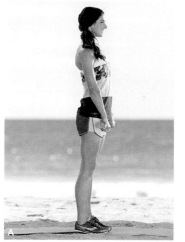
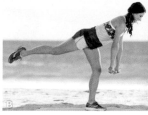
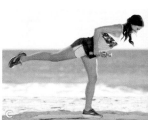

Circuit 1
One-Legged Bent-Over Row

Stand tall, holding a weight in each hand. Balancing on your left leg with a soft knee, hinge forward at the hip as you kick your right leg back behind you, maintaining a straight line down your back through your knee. Allow your arms to hang freely as you grasp the weights and row your elbows back, keeping them tucked into your side. Hold here for a count of one and slowly lower the weights back down. Repeat reps on same side for 30 seconds and then switch legs for a total of 60 seconds.

Single Leg Squat
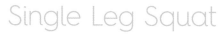

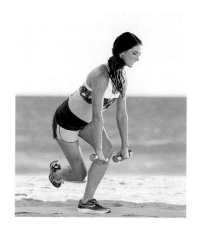

Begin by balancing on one leg with your core engaged, chest forward and shoulders back. Squat down bringing one leg behind you, keeping your knee in line with your ankle and behind your toes. Repeat as instructed, alternating left and right, for 60 seconds.

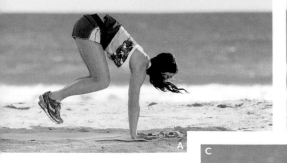

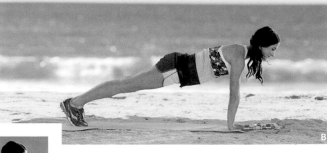

Burpee

Stand tall at the front of your mat. Reach down to the floor and place your hands by the outsides of your feet. Jump your feet backward to the back of your mat so that you land in a plank position. Hold for a count of one and jump your knees back up so that you land at the front of your mat. From here, adjust yourself into a squat position and drive down through your heels to jump up, reaching as high as possible. Land with soft knees and repeat as instructed. Do this for 2 minutes and then give yourself 60 seconds of rest!

Circuit 2
Standing Twist, Squat, and Overhead Tricep Press

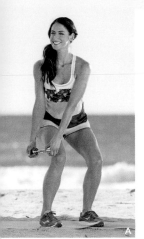

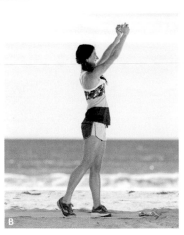

Stand tall with a single dumbbell held in your hands down in front of your hips. Perform a squat by shifting your weight to the backs of your heels and dropping your booty back and down. Keep your shoulders up and twist your hips to the right, touching the weight to the outside of your right calf, keeping your knees square. Press down through your heels to stand back up as you twist your hips to the left, bringing the weight across center and up overhead to perform a tricep press. Rotate your hips back to your right. Repeat as instructed, alternating left and right, for 60 seconds.

Bent-Over Row

Stand on your mat with a weight in your right hand. Balance on your left foot and step your right leg back behind you. Hinge slightly forward at the hips and bend your left knee to 90 degrees. Allow your right arm to hang freely under your shoulder with your weight in hand and rest your left forearm on your left knee. Pull your right elbow back and up to your side, performing a row. Slowly lower your arm back to the starting position. Repeat reps on same side for 30 seconds and then switch sides for a total of 60 seconds.

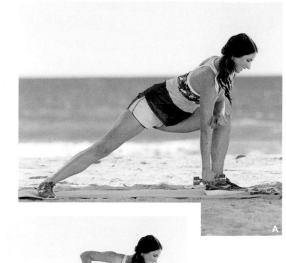

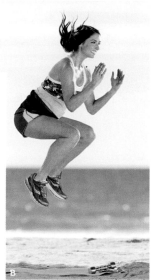

Jump Squat

Stand tall with your feet shoulder width apart. With a flat back, sit back with your weight in your heels and let your booty drop toward the floor. Make sure to keep your knees directly in line with your toes as you bring your quads as close to parallel with the floor as possible. Squeeze your abs as you press down through your heels and drive down into the ground to jump up, landing with soft knees. Repeat as instructed for 2 minutes and then rest for 60 seconds.

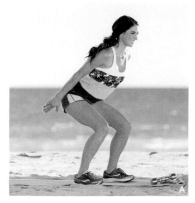

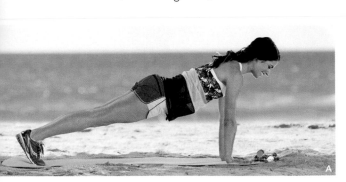

Circuit 3
Plié Squat, Twist, and Punch

Stand tall with your feet wider than shoulder width apart and feet pointed outward, holding a dumbbell in each hand. With a flat back, shift your weight back onto your heels as you let your booty drop toward the floor, allowing your knees to track outward to perform a plié squat. Make sure to keep your knees directly in line with your toes as you bring your quads as close to parallel with the floor as possible. Hold yourself in this position as you move your hands up by your shoulders, palms facing back, with your elbows down and tucked into your sides. Squeeze your abs as you punch your right arm across your chest, twisting to your right at your hips. Quickly pull your weight back to your shoulder, square your shoulders forward again, and then punch with your left arm as you twist to your left side. Pull your left arm back and square your shoulders with your hips again. Repeat as instructed, alternating sides, for 60 seconds.

Plank, Twist, and Kick

Align your body in a plank position, keeping your hips forward and core tight as you create a straight line from your shoulders through your hips to your ankles. Open your hips to the right as you pull your right arm up and extend it to the sky. Kick your bottom leg forward to hip level, keeping your foot off the ground. Hold here for a count of one and pull your arm and leg back down to their original position. Repeat as instructed, alternating sides, for 60 seconds.

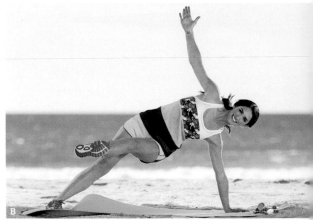

Plyo Lunge Jump

Stand on your mat and step your right foot out to lunge down as far as you can, keeping your booty back and your right knee in line with your right toes. Press down into your right heel and explode back up, launching yourself into the air as you tuck your left knee up in front of you. Land softly in the same lunge position. Complete reps on one side before performing on the other. Do this for 2 minutes, 60 seconds on each leg, and then rest for 60 seconds.

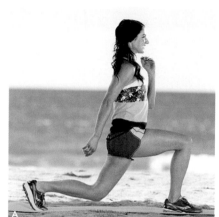
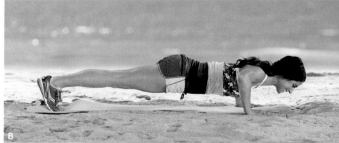

Circuit 4
Tricep Pushup

Align your body in a plank position, keeping your hips forward and core tight as you create a straight line from your shoulders through your hips to your ankles. Perform a tricep pushup by lowering yourself down with your arms, keeping your shoulders down and elbows tucked into your waistline. Once your hips are almost touching your mat, press the heel of your palms into the mat to rise again. Repeat as instructed for 60 seconds.

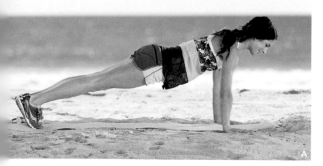

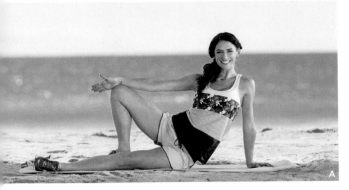
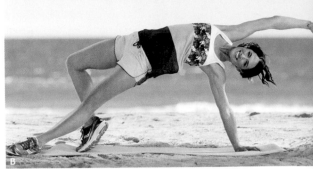

Rainbow

Come down onto your mat on your left hand and left foot. Stack your feet, place your hip onto the mat, and keep your left arm straight. With your right arm up above your head, pull your hips up off the mat, extending by lifting your hips as high as you can and allowing your arm to hang over your head. Hold for a count of one and slowly lower your hips back down to your mat. Complete reps on one side for 30 seconds and then the other, for a total of 60 seconds.

Mountain Climber

Come down onto your mat in a plank position with your hands stretched out under your shoulders, supporting your weight with your legs together and straight back behind you and your hips forward, squeezing your abs. Lift your right foot off the floor and bring your knee as close to your chest as you can. Return to the starting position and alternate sides. Repeat as instructed for 2 minutes.

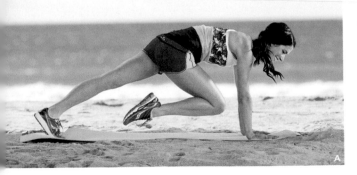
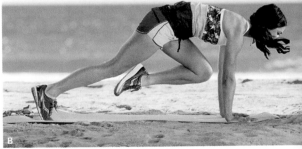

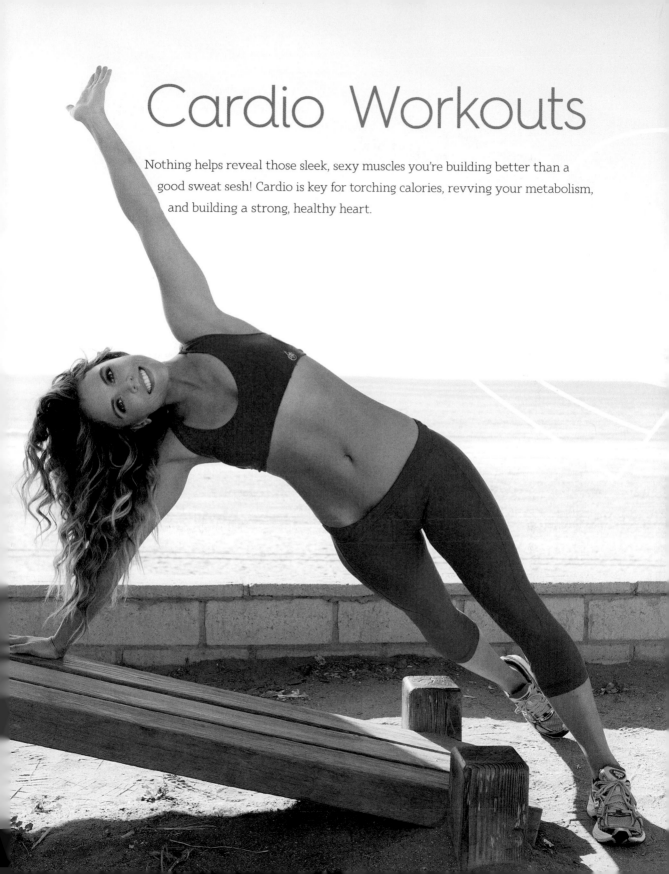

Cardio Workouts

Nothing helps reveal those sleek, sexy muscles you're building better than a good sweat sesh! Cardio is key for torching calories, revving your metabolism, and building a strong, healthy heart.

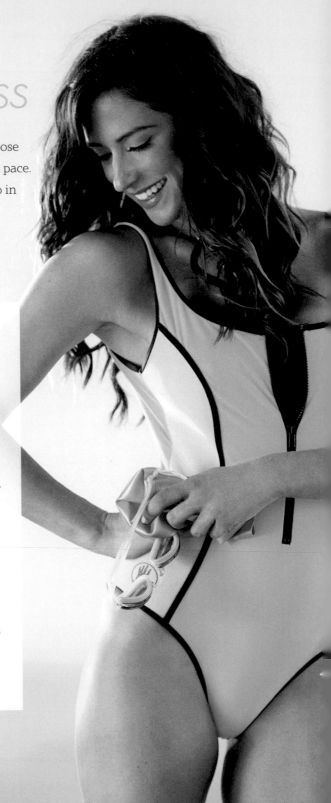

Go, Go, Goddess

This week we want you to just get movin'! Choose 25 minutes of your favorite cardio at your own pace. Run, bike, use the elliptical or stairmill, or jump in the pool for a swim. The goal is to build your cardiovascular base so that you gear up for the week ahead!

You know that feeling when you walk up just one flight of stairs and your heart is beating like crazy? I love when it happens for more than 40 minutes . . . on the stairmill! The stairmill is like doing over 1,500 squats in 40 minutes. It's pretty amazing for cardiovascular exercise, calorie blasting, and toning and lifting the buns.—Katrina

For a good sweat session, I love a nice long run on a hot day. Getting a workout done outdoors puts me at ease and helps me reconnect to myself.—Karena

2 Summertime Sizzle

This week we are building our cardio by upping the time to 30 minutes and adding intervals. If you don't have access to a treadmill, do your workout outdoors with no incline.

Walk/Run/Sprint	Incline	Time
Warmup walk	7 percent	5:00
Jog (6.0–7.0 mph)	4 percent	2:00
Run your heart out! (7+ mph)	2.5 percent	1:00
Walk (3.8–4.2 mph)	7+ percent	2:00
Jog (6.5–7.0 mph)	4 percent	2:00
Sprint! Push it (7.5+ mph)	2 percent	1:00
Walk (4.0–4.2 mph)	10 percent	2:00
Run (6.5–7.5 mph)	5 percent	2:00
SPRINT! Make it count!!	3 percent	0:30
REST! Carefully jump to the sides	2.5 percent	0:30
Sprint! You've got this!	2.5 percent	0:30
REST! Remember your goals	2.5 percent	0:30
Last sprint! GO GO GO!!	1.5 percent	0:45
Walk (4.0 mph)	5 percent	3:00
Jog (6.0 mph)	2.5 percent	3:00
Cool down (3–7 mph)	0 percent	4:00

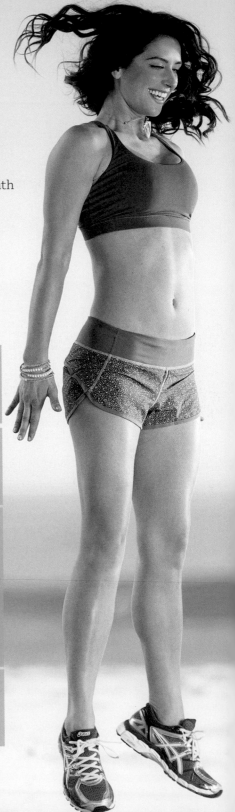

WEEK 3

Fly Me to the Moon

Ready, set, ZOOM! Here comes your 35-minute sweat session with the cardio of your choice. This week we are making our hearts even stronger by pushing ourselves to the limit. Use this scale to measure your intensity: Level 1–10 (1 = rest and 10 = all out!). You got this!

Warm Up	5-minute warmup (3–5)
Get Movin'	Complete the following 5 times: 30-second go all out (6–7) 1-minute tone it down (4–5)
Ready to Launch	Complete the following 5 times: 15-second sprint (8–10) 45-second Steady Girl (5–6)
Blast Off!	Complete this circuit 7 times! 15-second sprint (8–10) 45-second Burn Baby (6–7) 1-minute think about it (5–6)
Cool Down	3–5 minutes (3–4)

4

The Victory Lap

Bring it on home, baby! You're ready for an all-out 50-minute intense cardio session. We're using the same scale as last week (Level 1–10 when 1 = rest and 10 = all out!).

You have an option to do this once or twice this week. We dare you to do it on Day 23!!

3-minute brisk walk (warmup) (3–4)	60-second sprint as fast as you can (9–10)
4-minute jog (6–7)	2-minutes jog (5–6)

Chill for 30 seconds, breathe, and take a couple sips of water (take as much time as you think you need to calm your breathing).

30 plyometric lunges	60-second sprint as fast as you can (9–10)
4-minute brisk walk (4–5)	2-minute jog (6–7)
2-minute jog (6–7)	

Chill for 30 seconds, breathe, and take a couple sips of water (take as much time as you think you need to calm your breathing).

4-minute brisk walk (5–6)	60-second sprint as fast as you can (9–10)
3-minute jog (7–8)	3-minute jog (5–6)

Chill for 60 seconds, breathe, and take a couple sips of water.

30 burpees	60-second sprint as fast as you can (10)
3-minute brisk walk (5–6)	3-minutes jog (5–6)
4-minute jog (6–7)	

Chill for 60 seconds, breathe, and take a couple sips of water.

5-minute cooldown walk :)

Booty Calls!

Here's a collection of some of our favorite Booty Call options, to get your day started off right!

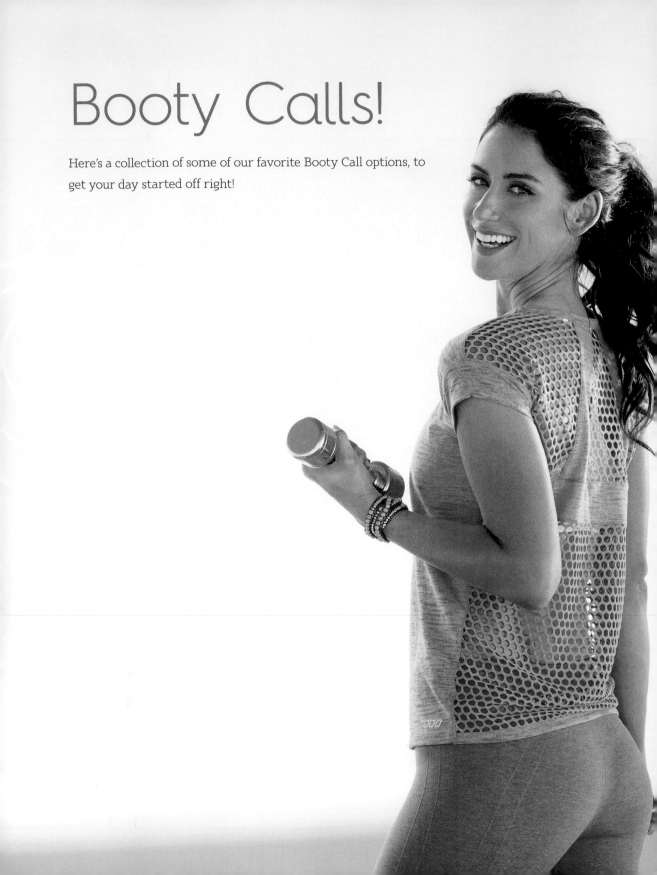

Amazing Abs and Arms

Feeling frisky and like you want a little extra love for abs and arms? Do this routine to build sleek limbs and a slender core. Complete three sets of 12 to 16 reps for each exercise.

Standing Twist and Uppercut

Stand tall on your mat with weights in your hands at your sides. Squeeze your abs and twist your shoulders to the right as you punch your left arm up, bringing your hand up to eye level, keeping your elbow under your wrist. Hold for a count of one and slowly lower back down to center. Repeat as instructed, alternating left and right.

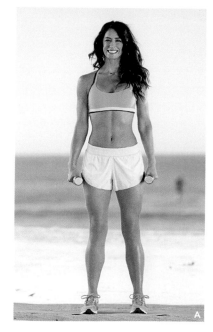

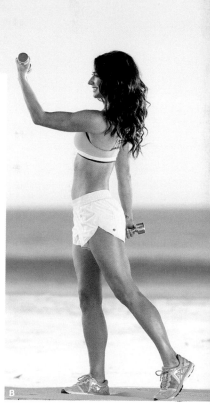

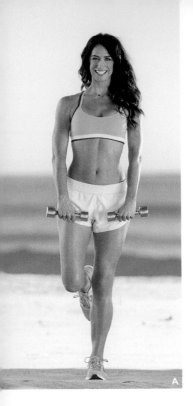

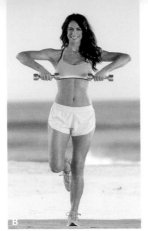

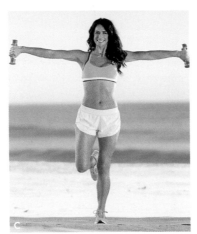

One-Legged Upright Row and Tricep Kickout

Stand tall on your left leg with your right leg behind you, toe on the ground if needed for balance. Grasp your weights in each hand and hold them at your hips, palms facing back. Engage your core and pull your shoulders back and down as you pull your elbows up to shoulder level to your sides, keeping the weights below your elbows (almost tucked into your armpits). Hold for a count of one, then kick your wrists directly out to your sides, extending your arms. Hold for another count of one and pull your arms back in to line up directly under your elbows, then slowly lower down to the starting position. Repeat as instructed, alternating sides.

Plank and Row

Align your body in a plank position, keeping your hips forward and core tight as you create a straight line from your shoulders through your hips to your ankles. Pull your right elbow back and into your side, rowing the weight while keeping your hips square to your mat. Hold for a count of one and slowly lower the weight back down to the mat. Repeat as instructed, alternating sides.

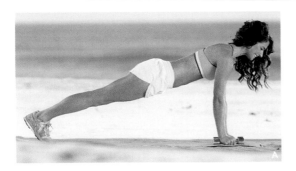

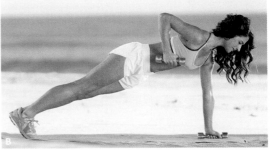

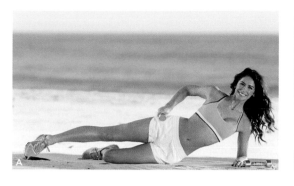 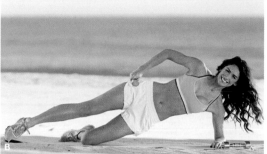

Dynamic Side Plank

Lie on your mat, resting on your left elbow and left hip. Stack your knees, pulling your bottom foot back behind you (keeping your hip on the mat), and place your right hand on your right hip. Lift your hips up off the mat, extending to lift them as high as you can. Hold for a count of one, then slowly lower your hips back down to your mat. Repeat as instructed, alternating sides.

Starfish Crunch

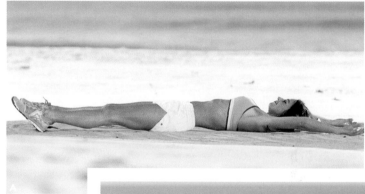

Lie on your mat with your arms stretched out overhead and your legs stretched out and straight, like a starfish. In one fluid movement, crunch your knees and shoulders off the ground and tuck your knees up to meet your chest, balancing on your booty. Reach around your knees to hug yourself and hold for a count of one. Slowly lower back down, reaching out in each direction with your arms and legs. Repeat as instructed.

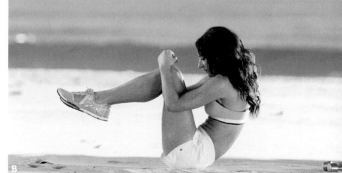

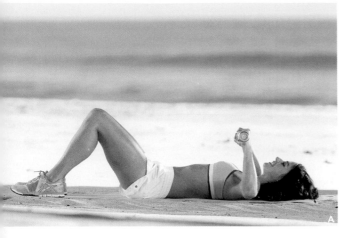

Lying Punch and Crunch

Lie on your back with your knees bent to 90 degrees, weights in your hands held up by your shoulders, and palms facing forward with elbows down and tucked into your sides. Squeeze your abs as you punch your right arm across your chest, twisting to your right at your hips. Quickly pull your weight back to your shoulder, square your shoulders forward again, and then punch with your left arm as you twist to your left side. Pull your left arm back and square your shoulders with your hips again. Repeat as instructed.

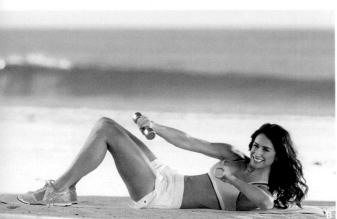

Booty Shorts

For a tight and toned tush, complete 1 to 2 sets of 10 to 12 reps each.

Lunge

Stand tall with your feet together and your arms at your sides holding two dumbbells. Step forward with your left leg into a forward lunge, keeping your left knee in line with your toes, and your left knee directly under your hips. Lower your right knee straight down to the ground as you bend slightly forward at the hips. Hold for a count of one, then press into your right heel to stand back up. Repeat as instructed, alternating legs.

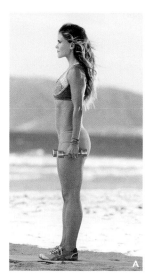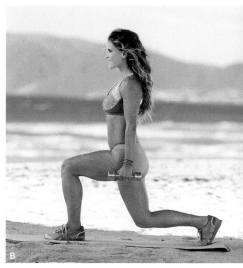

Standing Leg Abduction

Stand tall with your feet together, your core tight, and your hands by your hips holding your dumbbells. Kick your left leg out and up to your side. Lower your leg and repeat as instructed, alternating sides.

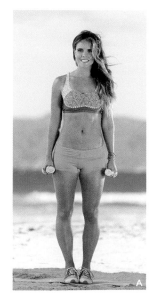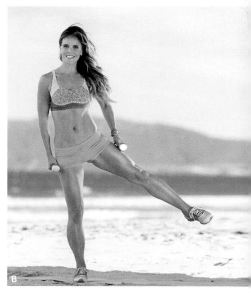

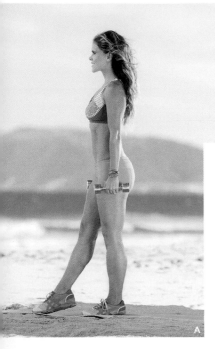

Pistol Squat

Stand tall on your left leg with your right foot a few inches off the ground and a weight clasped in each hand, held down at your sides, palms facing in. Squat back on your left leg by dropping your booty back and down and kick your right leg straight out in front of you. At the

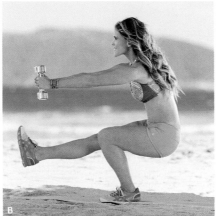

same time, raise your weights up and out in front of you, bringing them up to shoulder level. Lower yourself as low as you can—challenge yourself so that your left quad is parallel with the ground. Hold for a count of one, then press down into your left heel to stand back up, keeping your back flat. Lower your weight and your leg as you stand up. Repeat as instructed, alternating sides.

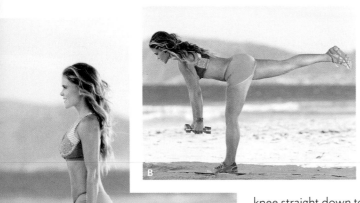

High Lunge into Single-Leg Deadlift

Stand tall with your feet together, arms by your sides holding dumbbells. Step forward with your left leg into a forward lunge, keeping your left knee in line with your toes and your right knee directly under your hips. Lower your right knee straight down to the ground as you bend slightly forward at the hips. Hold for a count of one. Then press into your left heel to stand back up, extending and lifting your right leg back behind you into the air and bending forward at the hip to bring your upper body parallel with the mat and arms hanging down. Hold for a count of one and return to your lunge with arms by your side. Complete reps on one side and then switch sides.

Weighted Glute Kickback

Come down onto your mat on your hands and knees, squaring your shoulders and hips with your mat. Maintaining a strong core, squeeze a weight behind your left knee. Lift your left knee off the mat and kick it back until your foot reaches up to the sky, making sure not to drop the weight. Hold for a count of one and then slowly lower your weight back down to your mat. Repeat as instructed.

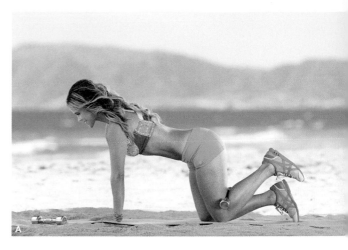

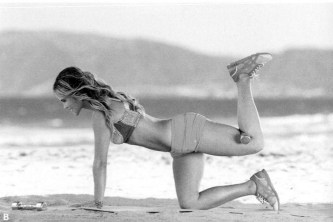

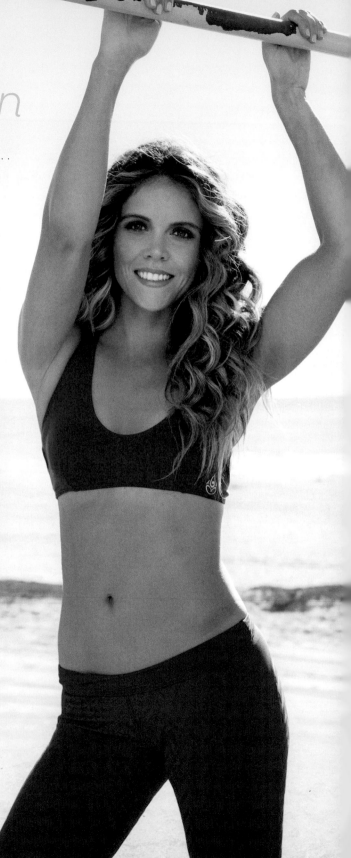

HIIT and Run

This HIIT workout can be done anywhere . . . and fast!

- 60 seconds jumping jacks
- 20 squats with a knee raise
- 30 lunges
- 20 pushups
- 60-second plank
- 30 plank jacks
- 40 bicycle crunches
- 30 lunges with a BOOTY KICKBACK! (when you come up from a lunge, kick your back leg up, toning your booty!)
- 20 squats with a bicep curl (use weights or water bottles)
- 60 seconds jumping jacks

Firecracker Intervals

If you're hitting the gym, try this heart-pumping HIIT routine!

Activities	Equipment	Time
Warmup	A machine you've never used	3:00
Hanging leg raises	Ab slings	3 sets of 20
Back extension	GHD (glute ham developers) machine or physio ball	3 sets of 20
Run your heart out!	Cardio machine 1	3:00
Squat and chop	Low cable	4 sets of 10 (each side)
Lunge and cable row	Low cable	4 sets of 10 (each side)
Run your heart out!	Cardio machine 2	3:00
Straight arm pulldown	High cable/ lat pulldown	3 sets of 20
Tricep extension	High cable	3 sets of 20
Run your heart out!	Cardio machine 3	3:00

Walk Your Way to Wow

Walking may not be sweaty or strenuous, but it's a great low-impact workout to reduce stress and boost serotonin. Walking is the perfect workout for when your body needs a rest and you want to set your mind at ease. Do this workout at your own pace on the days you want to walk but with a little pep in your step!

5-minute brisk walk
2-minute light jog
20 walking lunges
5-minute brisk walk
2-minute light jog
20 side lunges on one side and switch to 20 on other side

When we travel, we love to take walks to explore new cities.—Katrina

Repeat if you have more time for your Booty Call!

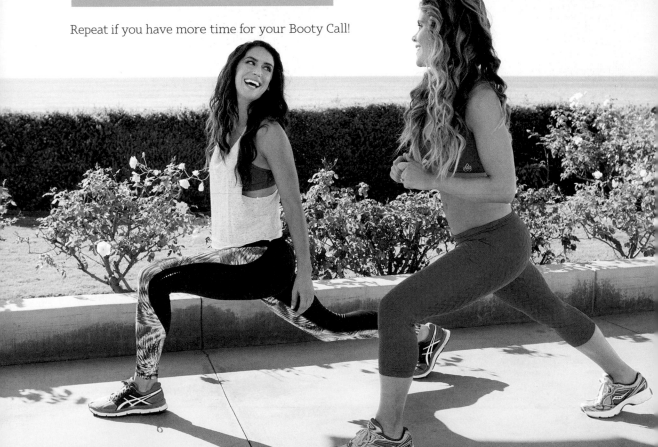

Yin Yoga

Yoga is one of our favorite ways to start the day in moving meditation or de-stress at the end of a busy day. There's something uniquely grounding about the mental and physical connection that you receive—not to mention the increased flexibility, muscle tone, and balance.

Cow Pose

Begin on all fours, palms on the mat. Stack your shoulders over your wrists and your hips over your knees. Inhale and arch your back, bringing your tail-bone to the sky as you gaze up. Immediately follow with Cat Pose (see below).

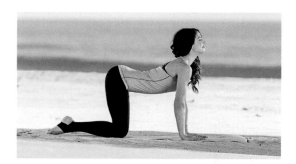

Cat Pose

From Cow Pose, exhale and round your spine by tilting your tailbone down and under and drawing your belly button up. Repeat the Cat/Cow combination 5 to 8 times to gently warm up your spine.

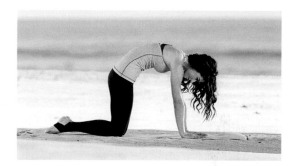

Downward-Facing Dog

Place your hands on the mat, shoulder width apart, palms flat and fingers spread wide. Align your feet so they are hip width apart, toes facing forward and your heels aiming toward the ground. Keep your spine long by drawing your tailbone to the sky. Leave a slight bend in the knees to protect the lower back. Hold this pose for 3 breaths.

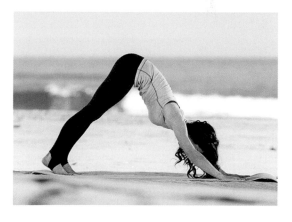

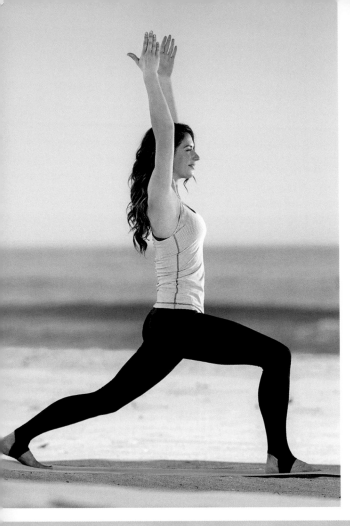

Crescent Lunge

From Downward-Facing Dog, step your right foot forward into a low lunge, the front knee bent to 90 degrees and the back leg extended straight behind. Both feet point forward, and you are on the ball of your back foot. Lift the arms overhead with your palms facing each other. Point your tailbone down, draw your shoulders away from your ears, and engage your core as you take three deep breaths. After the third breath, return your hands to either side of your front foot and step back into Downward-Facing Dog. Repeat on your left side, ending in Downward-Facing Dog.

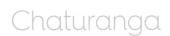

Chaturanga

From Downward-Facing Dog, shift forward onto the balls of your feet, coming into a high plank position with arms straight and shoulders stacked over your wrists. Keeping your neck and spine long and neutral, shift your body 2 inches forward. Exhale as you slowly hinge from your elbows to create a 90-degree bend. Holding your exhale, transition immediately into the next pose, Upward-Facing Dog.

Upward-Facing Dog

From Chaturanga, inhale and press your palms into the mat as you straighten your arms and drop your hips. Roll over the tops of your feet to shift your upper body forward, arching your back. Press down firmly with your palms to keep your thighs off the ground. Roll your shoulders down and back and lift your chest up toward the sky, then transition immediately (at the end of your inhalation) into the next pose, Revolving Crescent Lunge.

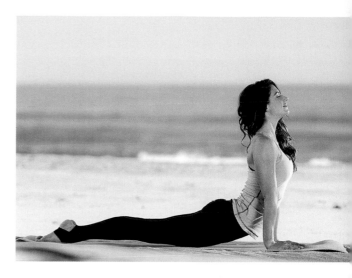

Revolving Crescent Lunge

From Upward-Facing Dog, push up to high plank position. Strongly engage your core to draw your right knee up toward your chest, stepping through into a low lunge. Keep your left hand on the ground while your right arm lifts straight up, twisting gently to the right. Your gaze is to the sky, and you hold this pose for 3 breaths. Then return your gaze and both hands to the floor. Step back to high plank, then Chaturanga, and return to Upward-Facing Dog. Repeat as instructed for your left side. After the second side is completed, press back from Upward-Facing Dog back to Downward-Facing Dog, to prepare for the next pose.

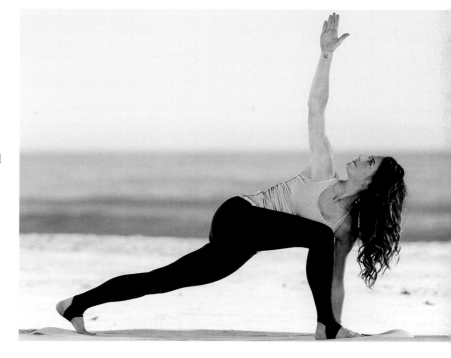

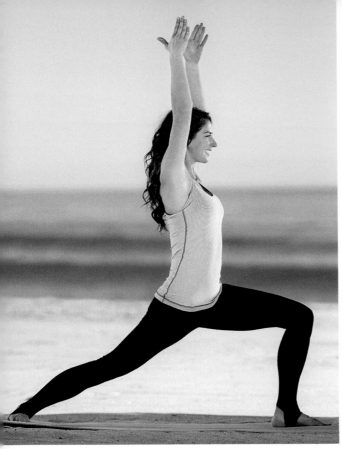

Warrior 1

From Downward-Facing Dog, step your left foot forward and pivot your back foot out in a 45-degree angle. Keep both heels grounded and your front knee stacked over the ankle. Reach your arms up high and turn your palms toward each other. Engage your core and remain in this pose for 2 breaths. Lower your arms and plant your palms on either side of your front foot, pressing back into Downward-Facing Dog. Repeat as instructed with the right leg forward, ending in Downward-Facing Dog.

Warrior 2

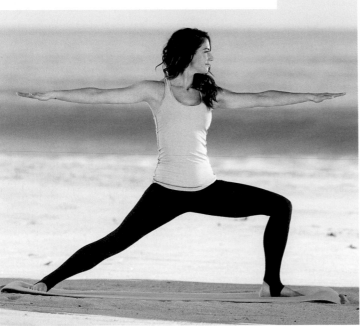

From Downward-Facing Dog, step your left leg forward into Warrior 1. Raise your arms as instructed for Warrior 1 for 1 breath, then extend your arms out to shoulder height, parallel to the mat. Tuck your tailbone toward the floor and gaze past your left fingertips (think Warrior!). Hold for 5 slow breaths, then windmill your arms down and bring your palms to either side of your right foot. Step back into Downward-Facing Dog and repeat as instructed with your right foot forward, ending in Downward-Facing Dog.

Reverse Warrior

Repeat the instructions from above to return to Warrior 2. Lift your front arm high and gaze to the sky as you let your back arm drop down toward your back leg. Arch your back slightly as you open your chest. Hold for 3 breaths, then return to Downward-Facing Dog as described above and repeat Reverse Warrior with your opposite leg forward. End in Downward-Facing Dog.

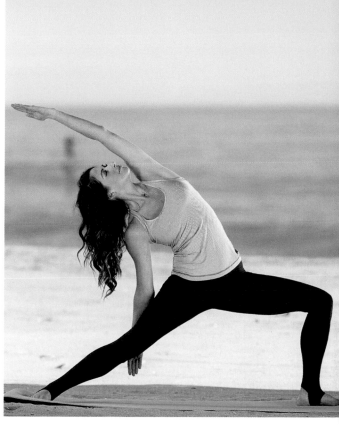

Extended Side Angle

From Downward-Facing Dog, repeat instructions for Warrior 2 pose, starting with your left foot forward. Bring your front arm down and rest that elbow lightly on the bended knee. Reach your back arm up and over as you open your chest and gaze upward. Hold for 3 breaths, then make your way back to Downward-Facing Dog and repeat on the other side, again ending in Downward-Facing Dog.

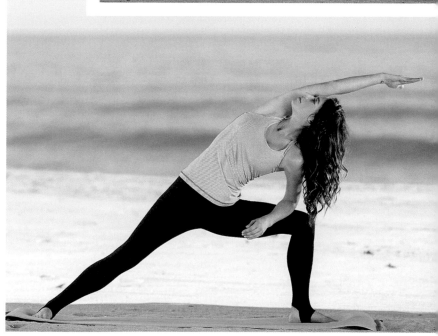

Triangle Pose

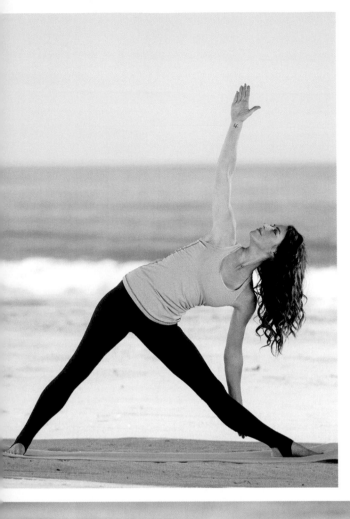

From Downward-Facing Dog, step your left foot forward and align your feet as you would for Warrior 2, but keep both legs straight (forming a triangle with your legs). Extend your arms as in Warrior 2. Shift your upper body slightly over your front leg as you bring your left hand down toward the ground, extending your right arm straight up toward the sky. Gaze upward at your extended right hand and hold for 3 slow breaths. Then, using your core, lift yourself back up to your starting position. Step back to Downward-Facing Dog and repeat as instructed with your right leg forward. End in Downward-Facing Dog.

Child's Pose

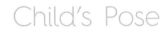

Bring your knees toward the edges of your mat and your toes together to touch. Rest your hips on your heels and sink your torso forward between your knees, bringing your forehead to rest on the mat. Reach your arms forward, palms facing down. Let your eyes close and end your practice by simply breathing, letting go of any tension. Namaste!

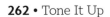

Resources

To learn more and join the Tone It Up community, visit ToneItUp.com. You can also find us online at:

Instagram @KarenaKatrina & @ToneItUp

Twitter @ToneItUp

YouTube Channel ToneItUp.TV

Facebook facebook.com/ToneItUp

To purchase Perfect Fit protein, go to MyPerfectFit.com. To shop all Tone It Up products, visit BeachBabe.com.

Acknowledgments

A big thank-you to our loved ones! Especially to our parents who have taught us to stay strong, persevere, and always keep following our dreams. To our loves, Brian and Bobby, who always stand by us. Thank you for your endless support and patience.

Thanks to the Tone It Up team who pour so much love and dedication into their work each and every day.

A special thanks to our agent, Eileen Cope, for tracking us down and telling us she believed we could write something wonderful; to our amazing editor, Marisa Vigilante, and everyone at Rodale Books.

And a shout-out to the rest of the incredible team that we couldn't have done this without: Debra Goldstein for her help in guiding us through the process of getting our ideas down on paper, and our talented friends and photographers John Segesta and Nicole Hill.

One last note of thanks to each other, for without the other, none of this would be possible.

Index

Boldface page references indicate photographs. <u>Underscored</u> references indicate boxed text.